Waking Up
from a stroke
The story of Crystal Jefferies-White

PETER MUIR

Cover by: Images With Impact

All rights reserved. No part of this book may be reproduced in any form by any electronic or mechanical means including photocopying, recording, or information storage and retrieval without permission in writing from the author.

Cover photograph by Brian Thompson republished with the express permission of The Brantford Expositor – Vibrant Magazine, a division of Postmedia Network Inc.

Available from Amazon.com and other retail outlets

Published by Images with Impact

Copyright © 2016 Peter Muir

All rights reserved.

ISBN-13: 978-0995037700 (Images with Impact)

ISBN-10: 0995037701

DEDICATION
From Crystal Jefferies-White

This book is dedicated to Jan Roadhouse, my friend, colleague and Speech Therapist. Every word that she helped me say was a key to a new and beautiful life. She has since passed. I give thanks for her life and work as I hope she looks down knowing how much I still love her.

Many people have helped me over the years. Those of us who suffer pain and loss can never repay the care-givers, neighbours, co-workers, family and friends who help us to get better. As we progress in recovery the list never seems to stop, but you know who you are. Please know that I thank you for your support and care. It is now my turn to pay it back.

INTRODUCTION

By Peter Muir

In my work at the Brantford General Hospital, I met and became friends with Crystal Jefferies White. I remember the news of her stroke shocked and saddened us when we heard that this popular nurse and friend didn't look like she would survive. I am happy to say that she managed to beat the odds, not only surviving but inspiring us as well.

As she began her recovery, I met her again at the hospital and was surprised. She was still the same bright, quick-witted person that I knew before but she was diligently working on recovering her speech. As I witnessed her daily struggles and successes I couldn't help but be inspired.

The day she walked into my office and explained to me why she wanted to write a book, it won me over immediately. Crystal has a way of gathering her friends together for a good cause and Crystal's determination amazes me to this day.

She was quite clear why she wanted her story told. Through this book, Crystal wants to help others who may be going through a stroke by sharing her experiences and tips to get better. She also wants to remind people that while the recovery from stroke can be painful, it can also include hope, love and laughter.

Both Crystal and I would like this book to be a useful resource for those who may have had a stroke or whose family member may have had one. While each stroke is different, there are some common challenges and that is why we have put in over 30 easy-to-understand tips.

Recovering from a stroke is a long-term event in a person's life. We hope that by sharing Crystal's story, from her early life to today, it may help ease the passage for stroke victims and their families on their way to recovery.

Waking Up

Waking Up

CONTENTS

	Resources	v
	Tips on Stroke	vi
1	A Spring Day	Pg 1
2	I'm Not Afraid To Laugh	Pg 7
3	A Wedding	Pg 15
4	The Making of A Nurse	Pg 22
5	The Conspiracy	Pg 29
6	The Rehab Conspiracy	Pg 43
7	Back On My Feet	Pg 51
8	Growing Up - Again	Pg 56
9	Recovery	Pg 63
10	You Speak Really Good English	Pg 69
11	Independence/Dependence	Pg 77
12	The Truth In "Giving Back"	Pg 87
13	Making A New Life	Pg 96
14	The Next Chapter	Pg 102

Waking Up

Waking Up

Resources

Aphasia Institute, Toronto

Rescue - Resources & Education for Stroke Caregivers' Understanding and Empowerment

Heart and Stroke Foundation

American Speech and Hearing Association

American Stroke Association

Stroke Recovery Association of British Columbia

National Stroke Association

Speakeasy Conversational Group

Dr. Thorsteinn Gunnarson

Hamilton-Wentworth Stroke Recovery Association

Lear Communication – Amy O'Connell

Tips In The Book

1	Aphasia Definition	Pg 1
2	Bell's Palsy	Pg 7
3	Visiting the Hospital	Pg 15
4	For Gatherings	Pg 18
5	Chronic Care	Pg 22
6	Swallowing Difficulties	Pg 24
7	Common Understanding	Pg 26
8	Preventing Falls	Pg 31
9	Levels of Aphasia	Pg 32
10	Socializing	Pg 34
11	For Conversation	Pg 37
12	Emotional Upset	Pg 39
13	Emotional Help	Pg 43
14	Rehabilitation	Pg 44
15	Occupational Therapy	Pg 45
16	Communication Alternatives	Pg 47
17	Medication Warning	Pg 51
18	Pain Management	Pg 53

19	Music Therapy	Pg 54
20	Try To Get Your Point Across	Pg 55
21	Speech Therapy	Pg 57
22	Conversation Ideas	Pg 60
23	Hint, Don't Correct	Pg 61
24	Phone Tip	Pg 63
25	Restaurant Tip	Pg 64
26	Changes In Vision	Pg 66
27	Consistent Crying	Pg 70
28	Humour and Stroke	Pg 82
29	Driving After Stroke	Pg 83
30	Driving and the Law	Pg 84
31	Chances of Driving Again	Pg 85
32	Volunteering	Pg 91
33	Fatigue Strategies	Pg 93
34	How Long To Recovery	Pg 97
35	Banking Tips	Pg 100
36	Divorce Statistics	Pg 102

Waking Up

1 A SPRING DAY

I am Crystal Jefferies-White and I feel compelled to share my experience with you. This is a real challenge because I have aphasia. I can speak to you out of my book, but if you meet me in person, my words come out hesitantly, as it is hard for me to find them. Sometimes they make sense and other times my attempts leave people with puzzled looks on their faces. However, I am determined, so if you stay with me, I can usually make you understand.

> **APHASIA**
>
> Aphasia is an acquired disorder caused by injury to the brain and affects a person's ability to communicate. It can seriously affect the ability to understand language and to talk, read and write.
> It most commonly occurs following a stroke.
>
> *Aphasia Institute, Toronto*

My friend and literary interpreter who has helped me to bring my story to you is Peter Muir. In our previous lives, we worked together at the Brantford General Hospital.
Why am I telling you my story? Mine is a story of hope. I am still here, coping, fiercely independent and happy to be

alive. Did I mention that I am not shy? During a portion of my recovery, Dr. Derek Dabreo, a Cardiac Specialist at the Brantford General, who is a good friend of mine, was shocked when he first saw me at the Brantford General post-stroke, saying, "Crystal, you are a real miracle."

Although he is a kind man, I knew he was being brutally honest as a doctor. Typically, patients with my condition do not survive. At that moment I realized, "that's the reason I am here." I have the chance to live my life one more time. Miracles can happen and I hope others can learn through my journey. Here we go.

TUESDAY MARCH 29, 2007

It was a typical spring day, full of promise, sunny and chilly, with buds just beginning to show. Since it was a beautiful day with the sun beaming down, I decided to sit outside and enjoy it. As I basked in the sunlight I stood up and felt dizzy, and weak on my feet, a feeling reminiscent of the first time I smoked a cigarette.

Stepping inside, the warmth of the wood stove permeated our old farmhouse. We lived in the country, in a community called Hatchley, just outside of the small village of Harley in Brant County. It was a lovely day so I decided to go inside and put some shorts on. I opened the door and that was the last moment I can remember.

Living with my husband, Jim, and my three sons meant that there was plenty of life, and fun, available. At 49, I was in the prime of my life and I loved it. On the other hand, as an RN, I knew how fragile a life could be. I had no idea that my life was about to change in an instant and I was about to awaken as a baby, reborn into a new life, having to learn to speak and write again. In a lucky stroke of coincidence, Jim was home that afternoon. Usually Jim worked during the day but that day he was home and decided to catch up on some chores around the farm.

Waking Up

My husband Jim White and I.

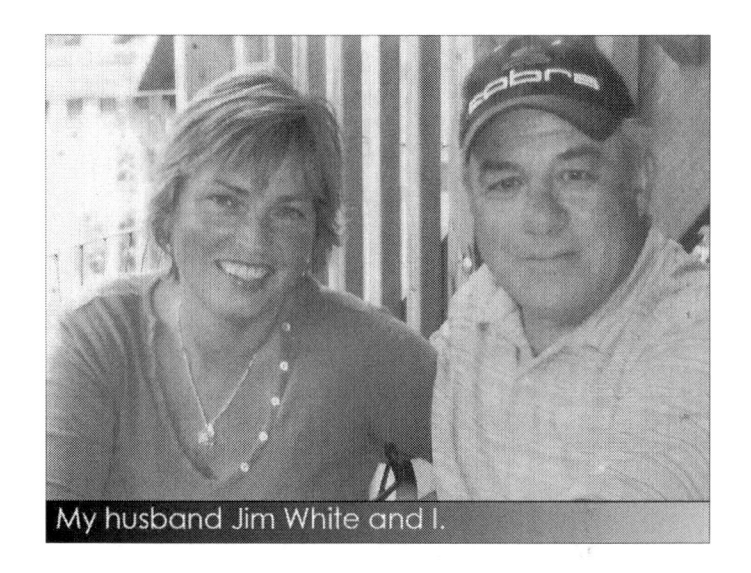

Jim came in and found me snoozing, noting that it was unusual to see me doing so in the afternoon. He slipped outside to continue his gardening. Thinking about me sleeping on the couch, he decided to check on me. He opened the door to find his wife - me - pointing to the vomit on the floor. (I really don't remember this). He went into the kitchen and grabbed a cloth to clean it up with.

Jim returned to his wife pointing to her mouth, trying to talk to him. With his wife unable to talk, he knew that something serious was up and called 911. He then made a hurried call to Kelly Lee our neighbor.

Following hard on the tails of the ambulance to the Brantford General Hospital, my husband got the bad news from Dr. Eric Irvine in the Emergency Department. He showed him the CT scanned images of the aneurism in my head, and the bleeding that was slowly increasing the pressure in my brain. I had suffered a cerebral brain aneurysm and a hemorrhagic stroke.

There were no appropriate beds available in all of Ontario so that night I was brought by helicopter to a

Buffalo hospital, the Millard Fillmore Gates Circle Hospital. This is an excellent facility known for its world-class neurological and stroke care. By 5:30 in the morning a team of doctors led by Dr. Levy had induced a coma and been able to coagulate the aneurism. They removed a large portion of my skull to give my brain room to expand, tucking it away surgically in my abdomen so that my body would not reject it when it was replaced.

Jim had a revealing conversation with Dr. Levy that he only shared with us later. He was told that "on a scale of ten with ten being death, I was a nine." He then sat in shock for the whole night and kept this information to himself so it wouldn't disturb the rest of the family. Meanwhile, my sister Kim was told that it was a hopeless situation with the best case being able to live in an assisted living home.

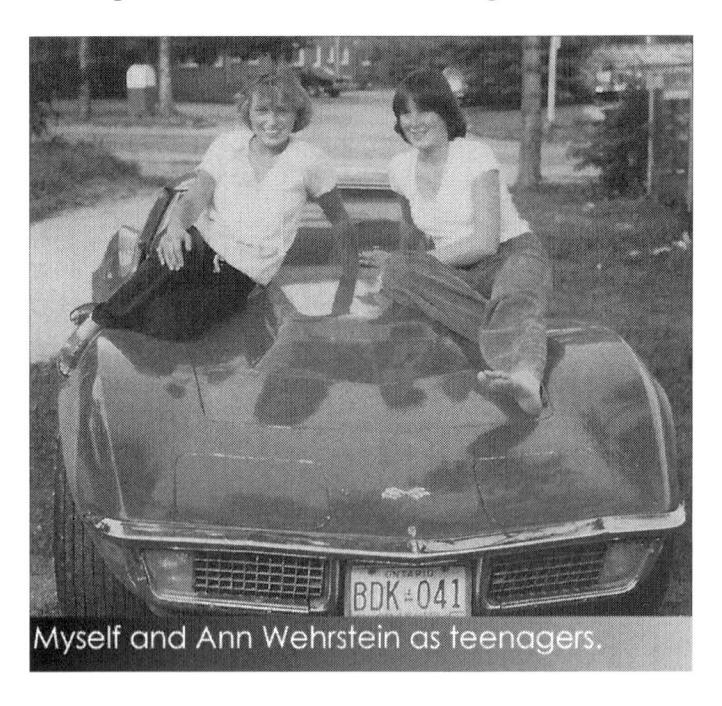

Myself and Ann Wehrstein as teenagers.

While I floated between life and death, I was watched over 24 hours a day by my sisters and Jim. My sisters Kim and Jackie slept over in the hospital room for the first few nights.

My good friend, Ann Wehrstein, when she heard about what had happened, dropped everything and drove to Buffalo to help out. She was of great assistance, helping my sisters cope with all the myriad details. My mother, Jennie and my stepfather, Nick were vacationing in Florida. When my mother got the word of my life and death struggle, Nick got her in the car and drove her back.

However, as the seconds became minutes and the minutes became hours, against all the odds, I continued to hang in there. Jim then waited for three weeks, travelling between Buffalo and Hatchley just watching over me while I remained in a coma and my body struggled to stay alive.

IN A COMA

There is life in a coma. Don't ever think there isn't. I know it first-hand. Through the fog and mist, it became crystal clear to me in one singular moment that encapsulated many moments.

It was a gradual floating I felt first. I was delighted to see my sons getting ready for a wedding. I remember distinctly the precision of the wooden archway and stained glass windows. There I was, floating again, feeling serene and then that sense of travelling vast distances in a second, a very distinct impression.

Lying in that hospital bed in Buffalo, I heard the voice of my niece, Logan and felt her rubbing my leg. My brother-in law, Billy, was standing in the doorway laughing.

I imagined my friend Ann and I were having a wonderful conversation about my son's wedding which wasn't to happen for years. It was all a wonderful party, yet it took place in one moment, in a hospital bed, in Buffalo. You know what I think? Time is just something we make up in our minds.

Waking Up

The strangest thing of all was this. I wasn't worried because throughout that evening, I could feel my hand being held by Jim and hear his voice. Another distinct image I could see was my dad's face. I knew he was watching over me. Don't ever think it is silly to talk with someone in a coma. We can still feel you and hear you.

2 I'M NOT AFRAID TO LAUGH

My life, somehow, has always been connected to stroke. In grade eight I came down with Bell's Palsy, a temporary paralysis of the face, which mimics the symptoms of a stroke.

The whole left side of my face ceased to function. It is a vivid memory, the entire 8th grade class laughing at my slurred speech.

I am not bothered by people laughing at me. It works for me and I even make a point of laughing at myself every day, regardless of the consequences.

Although I didn't know it then, that was my first taste of what aphasia could be like. It is very frustrating, as people may not understand you or, in that case, even make fun of you.

My teacher asked me to puff up my cheeks and I

> **BELL'S PALSY**
>
> Bell's Palsy is a facial paralysis that suddenly strikes all or part of one side of the face. Bell's palsy can appear with symptoms that cause many people to think they're having a stroke. In reality, stroke symptoms are quite different and Bell's palsy is a condition that usually clears up without treatment.

couldn't so he sent me home. My mother was a stay-at-home wife, and typically deferred to her husband on most matters.

Knowing this, I didn't want to show my mother as I thought I might get her worried, so I waited until my father came home. He hustled me out to the doctor's office who let him know what it was. Over time my face returned to normal.

Our genealogy is a mixed bag with the British, Ukrainians and Welsh all contributing their parts. My family

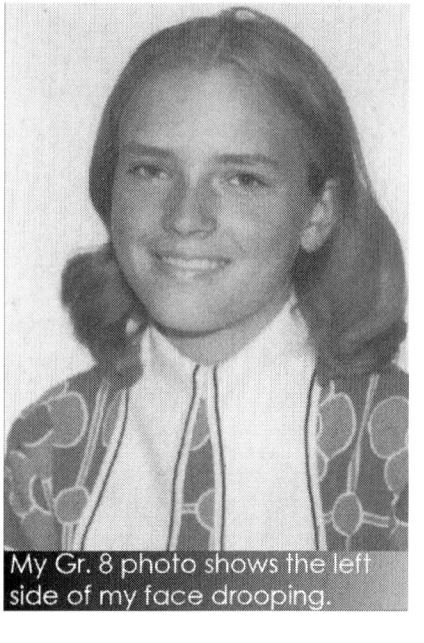

My Gr. 8 photo shows the left side of my face drooping.

started out with three girls, Kim, Jackie and myself as the oldest, along with my mother and father. Along the way we also picked up another girl and a boy.

Arlene and John had become friends with us as children and lived near us with their foster parents.

After staying late at my 16th birthday party they were afraid to go home as their parents were very strict. My dad felt for them and arranged for them to stay with us that night.

It was a turning point in all of our lives. In fact they now had a new home and are as close to our family today as any sibling can be. That incident sums up Garry Jefferies, my dad. My life changed that night and thanks to his example, I will always help others in need.

I hate to admit it, but I am my father's spoiled daughter, I was blessed/cursed with an independent nature and never hesitate to speak my mind. It is the same today. I am still trying to speak my mind, even if the words don't always come out right.

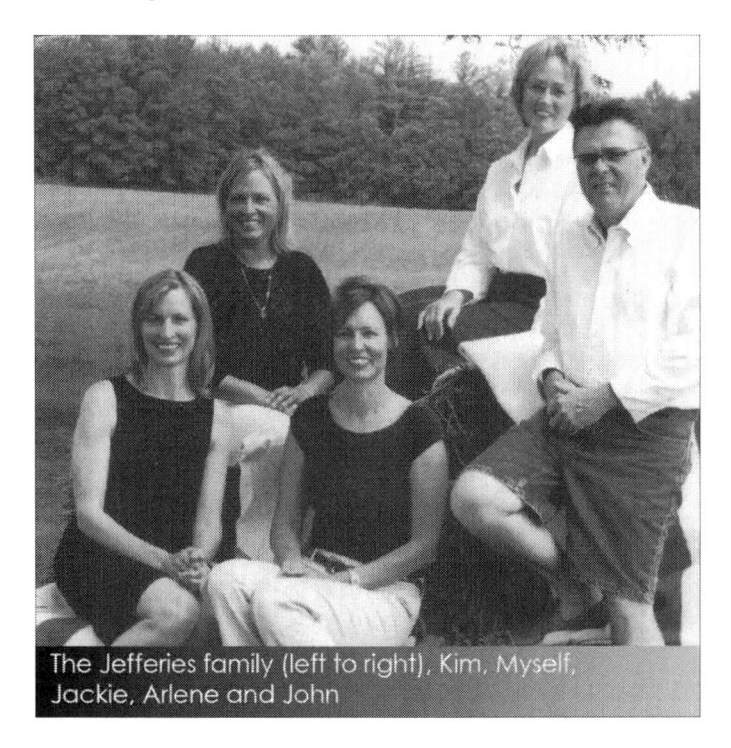

The Jefferies family (left to right), Kim, Myself, Jackie, Arlene and John

My dad was a huge figure in my life. After apprenticing, he worked hard to become the General Manager of a Lynden sod company, Fairlawn. My first job was cleaning my dad's office in our house. I was so thrilled when his boss, Bill Campbell, presented me with a cheque for $1. As an eight-year old at that time, it was an awesome lesson. Work and get paid!

The next hurdle for a girl stranded in the country was to get a license. Like many teenagers, and especially to me, it meant freedom. However, I found out that they don't just give away drivers licenses. At the time I didn't know that I would face a similar trauma later in life.

After three tries and despite some misgivings I

convinced the kindly Police Officer in Dundas to give me my license and have cherished it ever since.

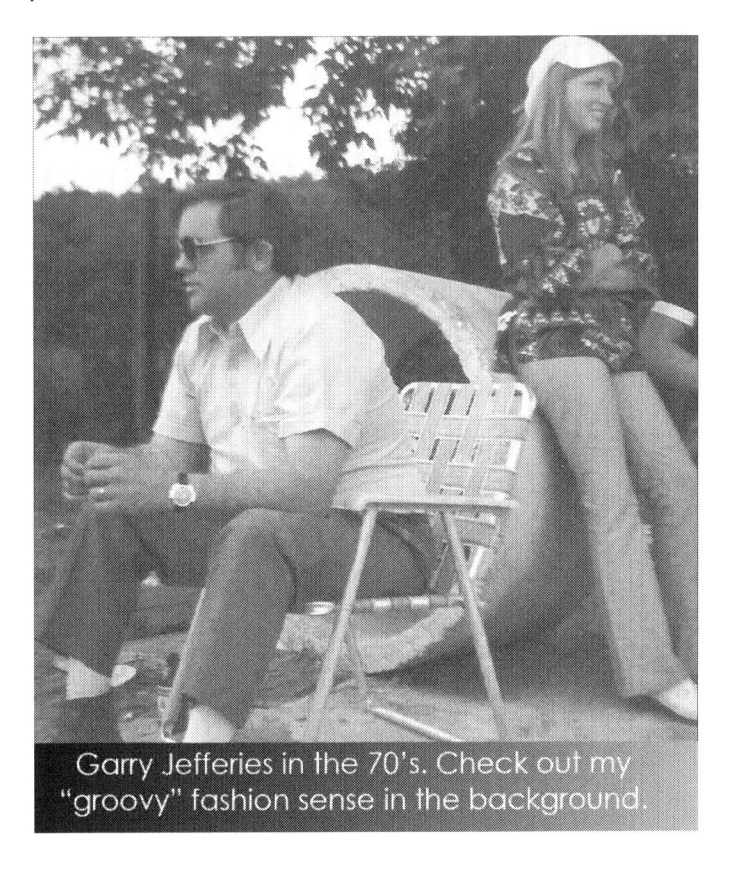

Garry Jefferies in the 70's. Check out my "groovy" fashion sense in the background.

Eager to earn some pocket money I got hired on as a waitress in a local restaurant. Waitressing is actually great training for being a nurse. It is where I first developed the skill of looking after five customers instead of just one at a time, a valuable technique for any nurse on a busy ward.

I was about to head off to work one morning when I heard the phone ring. One of my regular customers at the restaurant called me up out of the blue and asked me to work at his local hardware store. Ah, what you can accomplish when you are young and brash. My friend Gail needed a job just as much as me and I thought about how to get us both employment.

I was called in for the interview and brought Gail with me. To complete the weirdness of the situation, we were both dressed exactly the same. With a shocked look on his face the owner took me aside and said, "Crystal I called you, not your friend. There is just one job available." With the arrogance that can only come from a 16 year-old, I replied, "Well, I'm not going to be working here unless you hire both of us."

Gail was amazed when he hired us both. It actually worked out quite well for all of us. She worked there far longer than I did.

At a young age I realized that I am not a shy person. That is probably why I agreed to enter the Miss Outdoors Contest. Each high school nominated four students to take part in the contest. Now don't get me wrong, I love the outdoors, doing lots of snowmobiling and camping, but I wasn't really that interested in being "Miss Outdoors".

However, I could see the humorous part in the competition and I don't embarrass easily. As well, I couldn't let my sister top me since Kim was voted in that same year as, "Miss United Way".

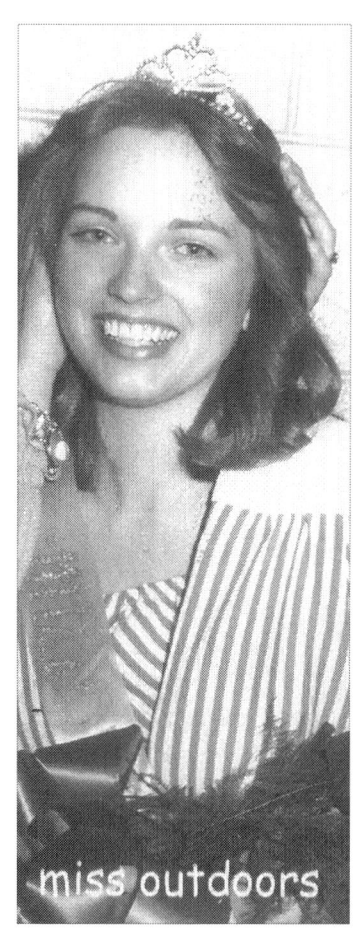

Waking Up

So when Terry Martin, the president of our student council approached me, saying, "Just do it. I only need one more girl to nominate," I agreed. When I won, it came as a complete surprise. It was the summer of beauty queens!

I had a natural talent in acting and one incident particularly stands out in my mind. I had taken a theatre class as an elective course and remember spending hours on my monologue for presentation in class.

The morning finally came. I was really nervous but also tremendously excited. When it came time to do my piece, I threw myself into it. It was a dramatic monologue and by the end of it I was in tears. The entire class fell silent. Then there was the sound of one person clapping loudly, my drama teacher. He followed it with a chorus of "Bravo!". I was pleased to find out that my efforts earned me a mark of 100%.

When I told my father that I wanted to be an actress, he laughed, looked me straight in the eye and said, "Sure, Crystal I always knew you were full of bullshit!" My father and I saw eye to eye on one thing. We "call them like we see them".

Knowing how insecure an acting career could be, he suggested that I come up with a backup plan in case my dreams didn't work out. That was the reason I ended up in the recruitment office of the Armed Forces one morning. To a young girl from a farm, the Armoury in Brantford was an impressive piece of architecture.

Surrounded by men in uniforms, the recruitment officer went through my options. When he suggested nursing, I was immediately attracted to it. However, only the Canadian Navy was training nurses at the time so he suggested I apply to them.

It wasn't such a wild idea. I wanted to travel, and the Canadian Navy would pay for your training while doing it. I looked into it and found out that to be a naval nurse you first had to graduate from a nursing school. My dad was delighted when I told him of my plans.

Honestly, I was a bit of a party girl at that time and as a grad nurse, I have to admit that I wasn't too attentive to my studies. I had a friend who was training to be a nurse in London, Bev White, who later took her husband's name of Thomson.

At the time I was dating a gorgeous fellow, John. He was a tall handsome, football hunk who had all the girls falling all over him. He was my first love. We had just broken up and Bev asked me if her brother, Jim, could give me a call.

The tall, handsome football hunk fell by the wayside as I grew into a full-blown love with my soon-to-be husband.

I admire Jim's honesty and his sense of fairness to this day, although, at times, I felt a bit sorry for his choice of a wife.

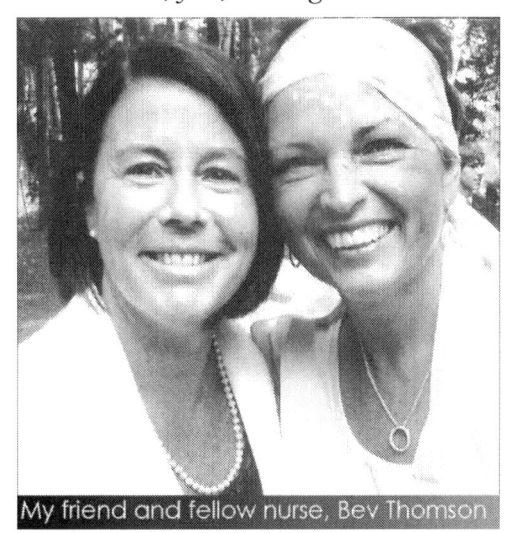

My friend and fellow nurse, Bev Thomson

FLOATING

I am floating again, and I'm quite sure that I am both a baby and adult at the same time. With great interest, I see below me an operating room in a hospital. The clinical setting is pervasive throughout the dream, with green hospital uniforms and ticking, humming machinery. A carefully measured, well-practiced familiarity is present in the surgeon threading the needle and turning to the patient.

Waking Up

With his assistant suctioning up the fluids with a long tube, the wound is closed and he begins with his needle, sewing sutures on her belly…it all seems very intimate and familiar.

Laying, shackled to my bed by IVs and breathing tubes, I slowly floated up and became aware of people around my bed. I could visualize their feelings, almost taste them. Jim, my sister, my sons, each wrapped up in their own anguish … contrasting with my immense joy that they were still with me. There I was floating again, imagining that I was talking to them…

3 A WEDDING

We all have heroes and my dad was mine. Our family has a joke that we bring out at family occasions – "Five teens - that's why my dad died so young!" Laughter sometimes helps to soothe the soul when you miss someone. However, when I think of my dad, I prefer to phrase it as, "Five teens – that's why my dad lived".

There's no denying it, my dad died young. He died when he was forty two. I was twenty one and he was the anchor of my ship. By that time, I was a nurse beginning my career at the Brantford General.

I got the sad call from my friend Marian, a nurse on shift at the hospital. My father had arrived at the Brantford General and I was to come

VISITING THE HOSPITAL

Nurses in Critical Care settings have to balance the physical needs of their patients, such as feeding, administering medications and medical appointments with their mental needs, family visits and rehab therapy.

At the same time they need to keep the environment peaceful and calm. The best strategy is to call the unit and talk with the nurse in charge.

quickly. Although she didn't tell me that my father was dead, I knew she was an experienced nurse and the situation was serious. Jim drove me to the hospital and the sad news came to me when I arrived. Our family was gathered together the Critical Care Unit and the tears in their eyes said it all. I was allowed to sit with my dad's body in the Critical Care Unit. It was very fast and he had passed away by the time I got there.

If you have ever been in one of these units, it is kept as quiet and peaceful as possible. The only sounds I could hear were those of the constantly alternating breathing machines and monitors in adjoining rooms.

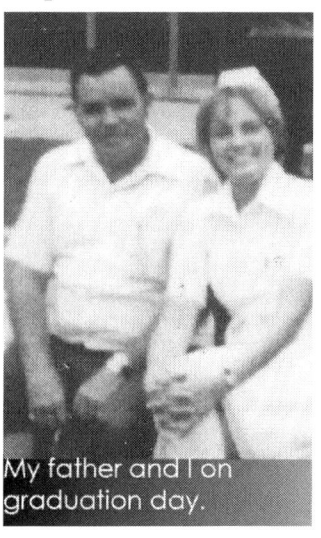

My father and I on graduation day.

As he lay there, my father seemed quite peaceful with his arms folded calmly on his chest. I watched his face closely. I knew at once that his soul had left his body. I looked up and said, "I still see you dad.". That is my last memory of him. In a hospital setting, we are always close to death and this was one of those special moments that the nursing profession has allowed me to appreciate.

Being the oldest I felt it was my duty to take charge of my dad's funeral arrangements. Despite what I felt, there would be no tears from me. I was determined to see it through to the end. I don't know why it stuck with me, but I remember dad relating to me the best kernel of wisdom he was given at his father's funeral, "He is happy now and wouldn't want to look down and see you sad." Good advice, I think.

Getting ready for the wedding with Jim along with beginning a new nursing job at the same time was a delicate balancing act. That was a tumultuous time for me and it was hard to cope with my dad's departure. When he died five months before the wedding, I couldn't help but take it as an omen. Discussing it with Jim, we decided to call the wedding off.

It was my practical Grandma Jefferies who put it into perspective and we managed to salvage our wedding. She pointed out that my dad loved Jim and was happy about us getting married. He would never want to look down and see that he was in the way of our happiness.

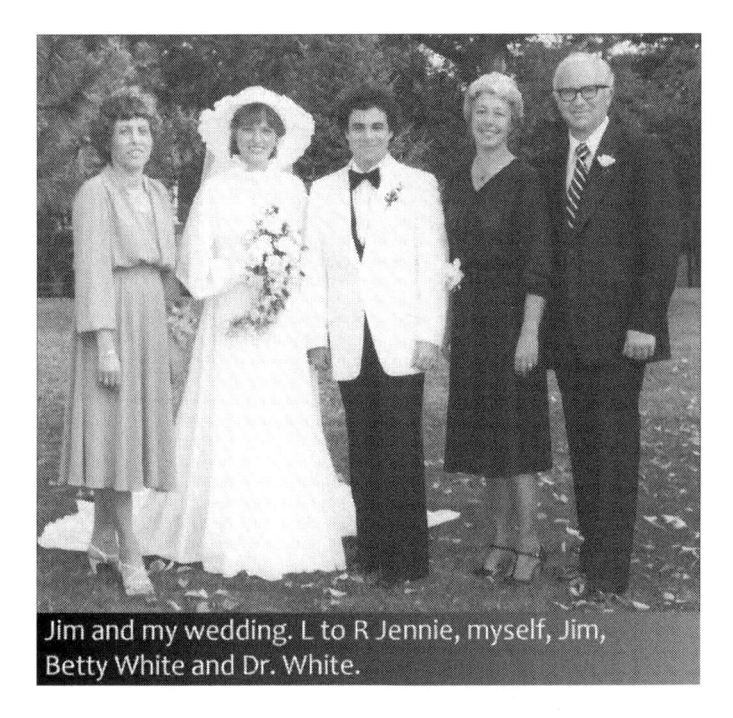

Jim and my wedding. L to R Jennie, myself, Jim, Betty White and Dr. White.

In fact my dad had already rented a hall and hired a live band before he passed away so he had an investment in the wedding. He was always a frugal man and I know he wouldn't have wanted us to waste it. We were right to go ahead with the wedding. Walking down that aisle with my Godfather Nick, I felt strong because Nick was on one side of me and I felt the spirit of my real father there on the other side.

It wasn't the fashion at the time, but I decided to part with tradition and keep my dad's name. I may have lost him but I was determined not to lose his name. When Dr. White, Jim's father, came to visit us after the wedding he saw the name tag on my nursing uniform and said, "Crystal, what's this?" I told him, "I lost my dad so I am keeping his name. I am proud of your name and that's why I took it." He smiled broadly at me and never questioned me about it again.

It was a great wedding and a wonderful honeymoon in Jamaica, but it didn't hit me until I got home. "I'm married to this man for the rest of my life." Our marriage together was a mix of dependence (I had a bit of the "spoiled wife" syndrome) and independence. However, despite our current separation, we are still always there for each other. That said, weddings have always been important occasions to me.

TIPS FOR GATHERINGS****

-Practice common things discussed in a variety of situations. For example, "How are you?" "It's been a long time since I've seen you."
-The more you practice this script, the greater your chances for success.

Later, when I first returned home, I was puzzled at the actions of my son James. I was convinced that he was married since I had seen it in my coma. However, he always stayed at home without his wife. I mentioned it to my friend Tracy and she laughed, telling me they had not married yet and were still dating.

Later, 10 years after they first started dating, they got engaged. I told my son, James that I would like to say a few words at his wedding but my husband, Jim, afraid of me embarrassing myself with my aphasic stumbles, insisted that I wasn't going to.

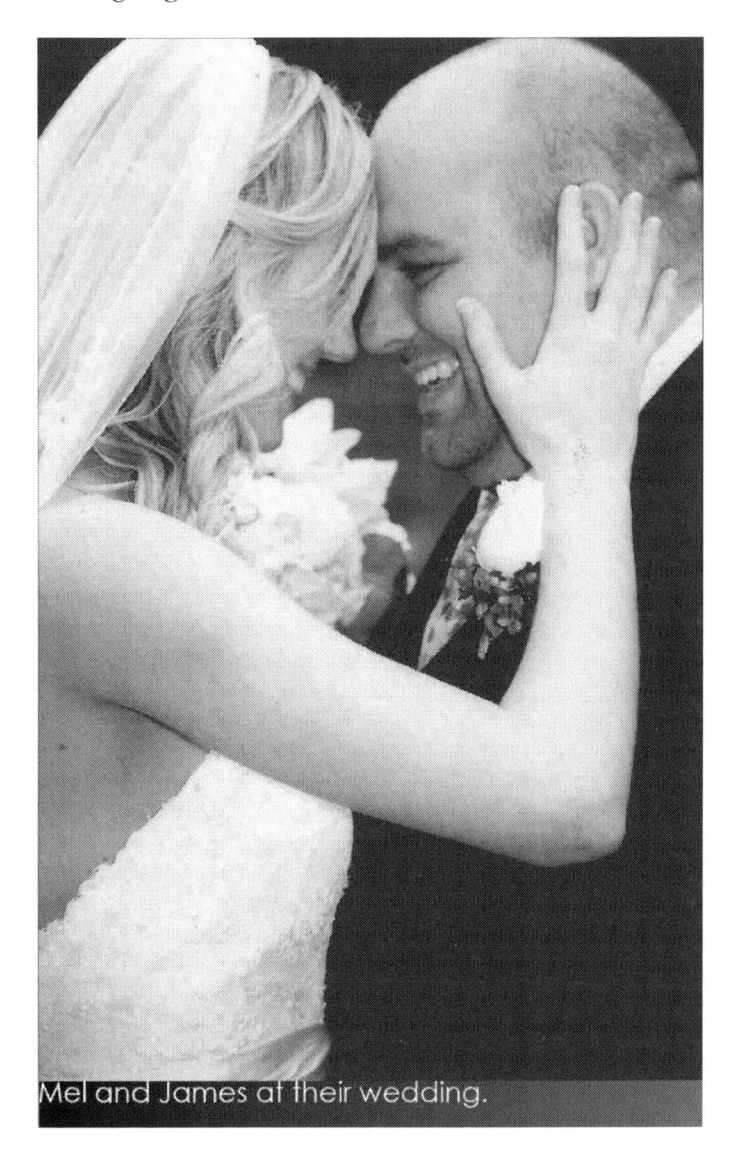

Mel and James at their wedding.

Now Jim and I have a very tumultuous but trusting relationship and we're not afraid to speak the truth. I looked him in the eye, very determined, and struggled to get out, "Just you watch."

Weeks before the happy occasion approached, we struggled with what I was to say. I had to really plan it out because nobody wants a sad speech at a wedding and I wanted it to also to be funny.

At the wedding, after rehearsing, and with Jim's help, I told people that, "James was seven pounds at birth, but now look at him." (Everyone knows that James is a big fellow.) I then told the wedding guests, "he has a heart to match his size." That seemed to sum my son up and I was proud because it succeeded in making the guests at the wedding have a good belly laugh.

A DREAM WEDDING

I was looking through the window of a hospital room. In the distance I could see a beautiful whitewashed church with colourful stained glass windows and a group of people gathered around it. The colours were incredibly vibrant like music to my eyes. They seemed all the more colourful knowing that there was an important wedding taking place.

Floating away from my bed, I came upon three men facing away from me. It warmed my heart to know that these were my three sons, all dressed in their finest suits. I was excited as they began to enter. I continued to float above them as they disappeared into the church. Realizing now that James was the groom, I was puzzled. "Did they rush the wedding because I was dying?"

Seeing them enter the church, I was so happy for my son and I could see a shimmering aura of love surrounding the entire wedding party. I hadn't even realized that they were engaged yet.

Everyone had filed into the church and I desperately wanted to follow. Even though I thought I was sure I was awake, for some reason, I couldn't move. I looked into the

Waking Up

church through the windows and saw all my boys lined up, coloured by the reflections of the stained glass, ready for the wedding.

The next moment I floated away, returning to my crib in Buffalo.

4 THE MAKING OF A NURSE

Miss Helen Baker was the head nurse at the Brantford General at that time. She had an excellent reputation as a top-notch nurse and was an even better mentor. I was fortunate to get a placement as a student nurse on her floor.

She was so supportive of me, insisting that once I graduated I take full-time work under her. It was too good an offer to turn down and although we had never met, the Navy and I regrettably had to part ways.

My first nursing assignment was on the stroke floor at the Brantford General. It was a chronic ward for people with stroke. Most had ambulatory problems, but quite a few people were unable to speak. Despite this, I could see in their eyes that they understood

CHRONIC CARE

A chronic condition is a human health condition or disease that is persistent and long-lasting in its effects or a disease that comes with time. The term chronic is usually applied when the course of the disease lasts for more than three months.

me.

Again, I would see stroke foreshadow my future life. My friends still tell the story of my first traumatic experience as a young neophyte nurse. I was caring for a stroke patient and had to feed him. I took my time feeding him and after a few bites he started to scream. It terrified me and I ran into the hall, yelling "Nurse!, Nurse!"

My friend, Marg Maker, a Registered Practical Nurse on shift with me came up and said, much to my chagrin, "Crystal, you are the nurse."

Returning to my distressed patient, it turned out that I was feeding him too slowly. With his communication challenges and my own inexperience,

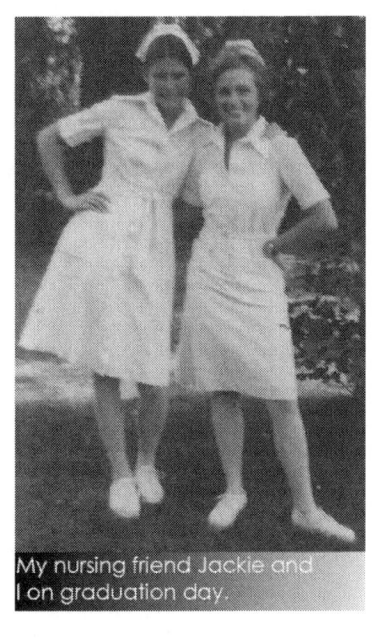

My nursing friend Jackie and I on graduation day.

he had no other way of letting me know. My nursing friends and I always had a good laugh about that one.

LEARNING ABOUT STROKE

It was a time of great learning for me. I remember the time that a nursing call light came on during the patient's dinner. I went to the room and there was a patient on the floor not able to breathe and turning blue. His fellow patient had pushed the call bell for him.

I began to perform mouth to mouth resuscitation on him but it felt like his airway was blocked. I called the ER and they rushed a team to my floor with a crash cart. The physician with the team quickly pulled out a large ball of food from the patient.

Stroke patients will often collect food in their cheeks and then swallow it, causing them to choke. After that experience it was the first thing that I would check for. I still remember the patient's first words after the team had left, "I want my dinner!"

> ## Swallowing difficulties
>
> Dysphagia is the medical term for difficulty swallowing or paralysis of the throat muscles. This can make eating, drinking and breathing difficult. Many stroke survivors experience trouble swallowing at some point immediately after a stroke, but this usually declines over time.
>
> Dietary changes may help with swallowing difficulties. You may be able to chew and swallow smaller pieces so chopping, mincing or puréeing food may make it easier for you to eat.

Another symptom is common among those who have suffered a stroke is the tendency to drool although it gets better over time. Once I took part in an aphasia support group. As a nurse I couldn't help myself and I remember going around the circle and wiping each chin with a tissue.

One of my first patients had a profound impression on me. He was an elderly stroke patient who had lost his voice, yet was only able to say one word, over and over.

Now, I can flash back to that hospital bed in Buffalo and relate to his experience. I/he didn't know that we had only one word. We thought we were talking in full sentences.

Every other week, this man had a special visitor, his friend, and mine, Walter Gretzky. Anyone who knows Walter will vouch that in addition to being a comic, he is a natural mime. Despite only having one word, I was amazed at how well he and this stroke victim were able to communicate.

When Walter left, I really felt for my patient and imagined what his life was like, not being able to express himself. Despite my empathetic feelings, never in a million years did I think that would ever be me. I think Walter and I may have felt the same way. A few years after his visit, Walter had a very similar stroke to mine.

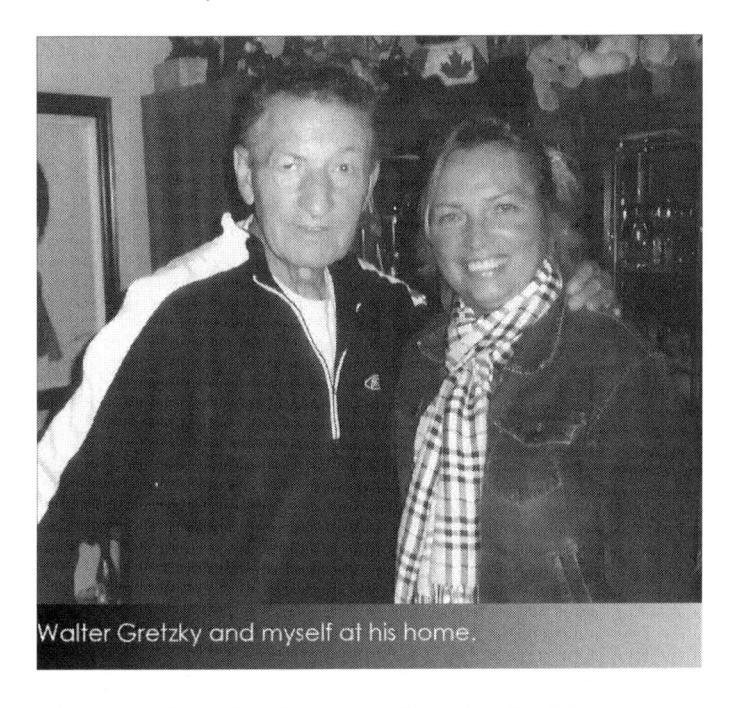

Walter Gretzky and myself at his home.

At that time, in the seventies, the healthcare system didn't recognize the special care needed for stroke patients. We just treated them as all other patients. Thankfully, our understanding of stroke related challenges have changed much in the ensuing years.

After many small strokes, Vera Jefferies, my grandmother, ended up on the floor of the hospital that I was working in. I was always fond of her. My dad's father died young so my Grandma raised him on her own. She was a pretty tough woman, earning a living as a correctional officer.

I have great memories of her. With her husband gone, Vera raised three boys and two girls, a huge achievement at any time but especially meaningful in the 50's and 60's. She was the best story teller and we grandchildren always made her read us her famous bed-time stories. Not having a lot of money, but eager to show us a good time, Vera often took us all camping and by the glow of the camp fire we would sing songs and tell stories until it was time to curl up in our sleeping bags under canvas. Great times.

> **OFFER UNDERSTANDING****
> Walter Gretzky himself suffered a stroke. Other stroke victims like Walter can support and understand what you have gone through as you talk about common experiences.

By the time she ended up in the hospital, her ability to speak was not affected but her mobility was severely restricted.

She didn't lose her spunk though, despite her weakened condition. I had to laugh when I overheard her tearing a strip off a young nurse, saying, "Don't you call me dear or honey, I'm nobody's dear!"

Before Grandmother Jefferies died, I was there every day, on my nursing floor, present at her side and helping her. That is one of the exclusive job benefits I have found in nursing. It exposes you to experiences others are not privileged to see.

TOUGH RESPONSIBILITIES

Nursing at that time paid well and I was good at it. That kept me at the Brantford General for five years until I

Waking Up

became pregnant with my son James. Returning from maternity leave, I was placed on part-time hours, a category of nursing employment which basically saw me filling positions all through the hospital. To help put bread on the table and supply equipment for three hockey-crazed boys, I also worked for the Victorian Order of Nurses, VON, along with other nursing positions.

One unforgettable incident scared me the most during my nursing career. I was a float nurse, which meant that I went wherever they were short nurses. This particular evening I ended up on the surgical floor. This is not a specialty that I was trained on and it was my first time on the unit.

One of the doctors called and ordered 1,000 KCL for the dosage of a drug in a patient's intravenous, IV. I wrote the order down and showed it to the charge nurse and she neglected to catch the doctor's error which quickly became my error. Not quite sure, I asked another nurse and they said it looked fine. I assumed the dosage was correct and started the patient's IV.

At the nursing station a doctor was reviewing the patient's chart and looked at me sharply, "Nurse, did you administer 1,000 KCL?" KCL is short for Potassium Chloride, a very powerful medication which

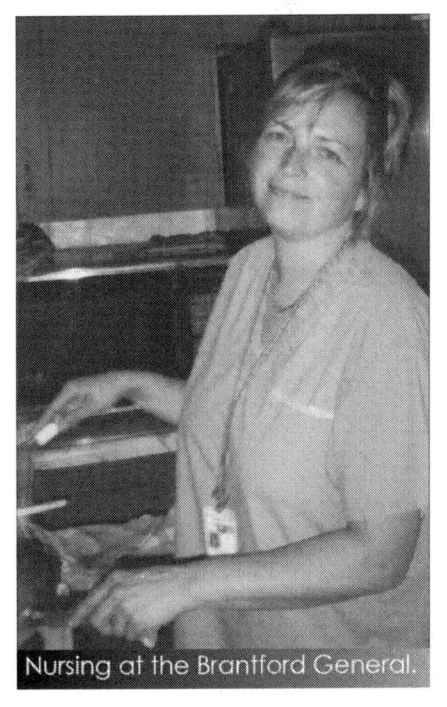

Nursing at the Brantford General.

must be carefully balanced or it can send a patient into arrhythmia. I said yes and he said, "that should be 100, not 1,000!"

While I ran to stop the IV the physician called the Critical Care Unit and the patient was whisked away on a gurney.

I was mortified. No nurse ever wants to do her patient harm. I began to cry. I knew that nurses should never assume that the medication is correct. I should have called the pharmacy myself if there was any question.

My friend Ann Wehrstein, took me into the IV room and showed me the labels on the cardboard container. She pointed out to me that it would have taken ten days to administer that much of the drug. Fortunately, it was caught in time and the patient recovered.

That night brought it all home very clearly and I advanced one further step along my chosen career path. While there are some awesome privileges to working as a nurse, there are some pretty tough responsibilities as well.

5 THE CONSPIRACY

Now that you know something about who I am, I will return to the story of my stroke.

I was a baby. I lay there in Buffalo, in a coma, and I was a new born baby. I could confirm this because I couldn't lift my head. It is a well-known fact that babies can't lift their heads and as an RN, I practice evidence based medicine. Curling up in a fetal ball, I indulged in this belief because it made me feel better. I even felt my dad hugging me.

At first, my son James had only one word that he said as a baby. "No, no, no". Strangely enough, I was told later that my voice became like a baby's and "No, no, no," was what I kept saying over and over in my baby state.

During my time in Buffalo, I remember crying like a new born baby. That image existed simultaneously to a scene that actually happened in the Buffalo hospital room, a combination of fantasy and reality. I was crying and my son James told the nurse to check the catheter. Sure enough, it was plugged. She fixed it and I stopped crying, just like a new born baby.

Even in a coma, there is some connection to reality. Laying in a hospital bed, I dreamt that I was in a crib. I was aware of the metal bars on the side and the large headboard and footboard, but preferred to indulge in my baby fantasy.

Waking Up

To me, it was my crib.

I felt a pain in my chest, exactly like someone was squeezing it and I made whimpering noises just like a baby. When I described it later, after coming out of the coma, my son was amazed since Dr. Levy had squeezed me there as a test of responsiveness while in the coma.

I remember distinctly laying in my hospital bed… then travelling back in time and beginning the long fall down the stairs in my stroller as a toddler, and then I was up, floating as a baby again.

It took me a while to wake up. As I slowly climbed out of the induced coma in Buffalo the world didn't seem any more solid than my illusory world of dreams. The world I woke up in was filled with conspiracies. It all began in Buffalo. I was convinced that the staff were keeping me drugged to imprison me in the hospital.

One night, as the nurse changed the IV bag, I pretended to be asleep. When she left the room I struggled to reach the IV and pull it out. This went on through my imprisonment. They tell me that I succeeded in pulling it out occasionally.

They couldn't fool me. There was one nurse that seemed to be the main villain. She was the one poisoning me and I was deathly afraid anytime she would enter the room. Later, Jim would concur with me and say he was afraid of her too. I think his reasoning and mine were probably very different.

Tied to the tubes and restrained in the bed, I was convinced that I was a prisoner. Half in and out of a coma, I screamed for them to let me go. As a result of my screaming the nurse who I suspected was poisoning me had me moved into a private room and gave me a dose of something to settle me. I thought it had Gravol in it since I began drifting off to sleep. Now I knew she was poisoning me.

That night, I pulled Jim to my side and whispered, "Jim, Jim, get me out of here. That nurse is killing me." Jim nodded and a moment later the patient transport personnel came to get me. I was thrilled since Jim had obviously understood me (or I thought he did). Although it seemed like a coincidence in retrospect, I don't believe in coincidences.

Jim brought me to Canada and the Hamilton General Hospital in the ambulance. I felt safer there. Peaceful, and relaxed, my memory started to become clearer. No more screaming.

HAMILTON GENERAL HOSPITAL

Although I didn't quite seem myself yet, I was desperate to communicate. Jim remembers me trying to use the palm of his hand as a cell phone. When I did get him to call people for me, I would get on the phone and talk incessantly. In my mind what I was saying all made sense.

> **PREVENT FALLS*****
>
> Statistics show that 40 percent of all stroke survivors suffer serious falls within a year after their stroke.
> It will help if you:
>
> -Clear paths to the kitchen, bedroom and bathroom
> -Remove loose carpets and runners in hallways and stairwells, or fasten them with nonskid tape
> -Install handrails for support in going up and down stairs

I was really unsteady on my feet still. One day I had to go to the washroom and pushed the call bell. Trying it a number of times with no response I waited. After a few minutes with no care-giver in sight, I decided to take care of it myself.

Struggling to get the bed rail down I pushed myself out of the hospital bed. The first couple of steps were manageable but I could feel how unsteady I was. Quickly grabbing the doorway to steady myself, I managed to complete my business. I remember thinking with my nurses cap on, "so that is how falls happen." Take note nurses, how important it is to answer call bells!

I remember looking at my arms and then my legs in the Hamilton General. You could see the tone and definition of my muscles and I marveled at how slim they were, thinking, "They're looking really good."

Then the awful reality of the situation set in and stuck to me like a mental burr – I was losing weight and dying of cancer. Now I understood. As a nurse I diagnosed all the symptoms and it was an irrefutable fact. I was dying of this dreadful disease.

Everybody seemed to be in on the cover-up. I realized that Jim was just going to deny it, to try and give me hope and keep my spirits up. I wondered who else was in on the secret.

The fact that I had terminal cancer explained something that had been bothering me. Every time I talked to someone they would just nod and smile at me. They were feeling sorry for me and afraid to upset me. That was it! It was a grand conspiracy.

So I asked my family whether I was dying of cancer (or I thought I was asking them if I was dying of cancer). My suspicions were confirmed when no-one disagreed with me. However, bless their hearts, my friends and family kept trying to help me understand the truth.

LEVELS OF APHASIA *****

Aphasia can be so severe as to make communication with the person extremely challenging. Occasionally it affects only a single aspect of language, such as the ability to read.

Waking Up

Lucidity was coming to me slowly. That same day, my father-in-law, Dr. White and his wife came to visit me. He sat there watching me and not talking. I decided to start a conversation with him and did so. It all sounded fine to me as I asked him how he was feeling.

He turned to his wife and said, "What did she call me?" That is when I realized there was a problem. I then knew that what my head thought and my mouth said were not necessarily the same. I just wasn't speaking right. I knew who Dr. White was but another word had obviously come out of my mouth.

However, as a "trained" nurse, I was certain that this lack of understanding was obviously a strange symptom caused by my cancer symptoms and I just had to get through it.

MY TERMINAL ILLNESS

People can be so nice. Although my words made perfect sense in my head, in reality I was talking gibberish to my loved ones. Not wanting to disturb me, they would laugh and pretend to understand me. No-one corrected me.

Even though I was on death's door as a terminal cancer patient, I refused to give in to tears. Except once. My son, Jared had come to visit me with Jim. My attitude towards raising children has always been to try and protect them from life's difficulties and not be dependent on them.

That is why I told Jared to go home and Jim to stay. In my fuzzy mental state, I wasn't able to understand the fact that they had come together in the same vehicle and had to leave together.

When they left the room I thought Jim was just seeing Jared off and would be back. After a while I realized that Jim would not be coming back and I thought it was proof that he didn't care. That was the one time I did cry.

In my eyes, that act made Jim the focus of the

conspiracy. He was to blame for almost everything amiss. For example, I had inherited my dad's ring after he died and it was always a treasure of mine until it disappeared in Buffalo. A gold ring, I was convinced that Jim had slipped it off my finger and sold it.

The big day finally came though. It was my first pass from the hospital and I was finally allowed to leave Hamilton. Maybe, just maybe, I didn't have cancer and I would go home, wake up one day and have my words back.

On the way back home from Hamilton, Jim was driving and my sister, Kim was sitting in the back seat. Seated in the passenger side, I was feeling very isolated and alone, not able to follow their conversation. They began referring to me as if I wasn't present in the car.

That was a really long ride back. I just stared out the window, thinking, "Do you think I am simple? My mind works perfectly; I am just not able to speak." I was very frustrated with my newly-discovered condition.

Socializing*****

For many survivors, this loss or change in speech and language profoundly alters their social life.

-Ironically, research has shown that socializing is one of the best ways to maximize stroke recovery.
-Many experts contend that socializing should begin right away in the recovery process.

When I spied a road sign for Hatchley, I was happy. Up until then I had no idea where I was. Arriving back at the farmhouse, my entire family, both sides of them and a goodly portion of my friends were waiting. I sat with them, not talking because I couldn't be understood or understand. I was just watching them, laughing, having a good time, no tears among the bunch. It became obvious that they all were just covering up their true feelings, knowing I had cancer.

I sat there in my kitchen, so intimately familiar to me, not speaking, not being able to speak and not understanding it when I heard the conversation. It all started quietly, me... sitting there in silence. Slowly out of the corner of my eye, one tear rolled out, inexorably followed by another and then another. The attitude of my family changed in that moment – we all began crying. Inside, I was relieved and happy, knowing that they didn't have to pretend anymore. They could now acknowledge that I was dying of cancer.

HAMILTON

At the Hamilton General Hospital the news wasn't good. They had discovered another aneurysm in my brain that had not burst. Dr. Kalirfan arranged to do a major surgery to repair my brain. In Buffalo they had repaired the aneurysm in the left middle cerebral artery and that one was still stable.

Dr. Thorsteinn Gunnarson, my neurologist at the Hamilton General describes an aneurysm as a "blister on the artery," and this one was threatening to burst. So I went under the anaesthetic again on December 18 of 2008. This operation was to be on my anterior communicating artery.

In the Hamilton General Hospital, Jim's sister, Bev had to help me into the bathroom since I was still unsteady. It was the first time that I looked in the mirror since awakening.

There was a definite dint in the left side of my skull. I touched it in amazement. Bev then showed me the fresh scar on my belly. I gasped. While floating in a coma, I had seen the surgeon carefully placing that piece of skull in an abdomen. At the time I had no idea it was mine. I felt the scar in my head and realized that I was the patient on the gurney.

As I began to recover, they allowed me out on a two-day pass. Occasionally, I was able to say a couple of words such as "No, No, No," and "Me, me, me," but was still having trouble connecting my brain to what I said. I didn't even realize that the words were coming out all wrong. I got the idea, though when Dr. White visited me and repeated what I was saying. It was a hard realization.

However, In all my confusion, there was a breakthrough one weekend.

BULL-SHIT!

Jim, Kelly, Brian and I sat on the back deck in Hatchley overlooking the growing corn in the field. I had a flash-back to the time my dad looked me in the eye when I told him I wanted to be an actor and what he said that evening.

As we sat on the porch, I felt frustrated and confused. At the hospital visitors either laughed cheerfully or cried when they saw me. I felt like I was a living funeral.

Here we were on the back porch of my own home and it was like nothing had changed, although so much had. As on many Friday nights in the past, our neighbours, Kelly and Brian visited us to enjoy the evening on the back porch.

I tried to listen to the conversation but I could barely understand what these people, who were my friends and loved ones, were talking about. Yet they acted as if I was the same person, with the same understanding.

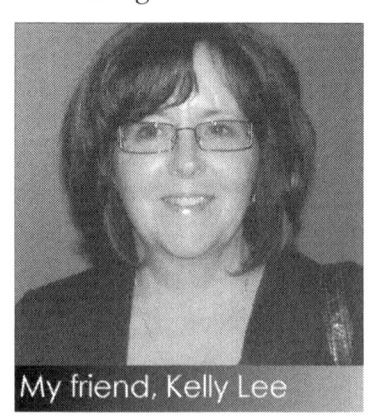

Jim teased me as usual, but that day, in Hatchley, back at

my own home - I couldn't defend myself, I had changed. I sat there furious, emotions boiling. How could my own husband not see how I was feeling?

Without any prompting or forethought, the word just leaped out of my mouth..."BULLSHIT!"

It was a cathartic moment that changed my attitude. It was the first two syllable word that I uttered since my awakening. My dad would have been proud. After a moment of shocked silence, Jim burst out in laughter, followed by Kelly and Brian. We all laughed and the anger and frustration flew away. I had said something else! I turned my gaze upward and thought of the fellow who started it all. Thanks Dad.

Although I couldn't repeat it after that incident, Kelly and I worked on it until I became fluent in Bullshit again. It's good to have a friend like Kelly as this isn't the kind of thing they teach you in speech therapy.

Although it isn't discussed in many stroke manuals, a sure sign of my recovery was the day I realized that Jim and I were yelling at each other angrily. We had that kind of relationship prior to my stroke and the fact that we were back to our everyday ways was yet another sign that I was healing.

CONVERSATION*****

It is easiest to begin practicing conversation in a one-on-one situation with someone comfortable, who understands your communication disorder.

THE GROUP HOME CONSPIRACY

My greatest fear was going to that dreaded assisted living group home. At this stage in my recovery, I was still not clear on what people were saying to me.

I had convinced myself that I heard Jim talking about putting me in a group home. I thought I overheard him say the word, "oxygen", and the awful truth fell into place, It was lung cancer! I was stricken with deadly lung cancer.

It all made sense. I knew it was the most common cause of cancer. I thought guiltily of how we would smoke every time I participated in the nurses' weekend. These were particularly wild times we had at my friend, Marlyn's cottage. Twice a year she invited a bunch of us nurses up to her place to shop and party. You know us nurses, work hard and play hard!

I thought that I had dodged that bullet when I quit smoking full-time twenty years ago, with my first pregnancy. There it was. My sinful past coming back to haunt me. I always knew that cigarettes are like Russian Roulette - the bullet could strike anyone and my number had just come up.

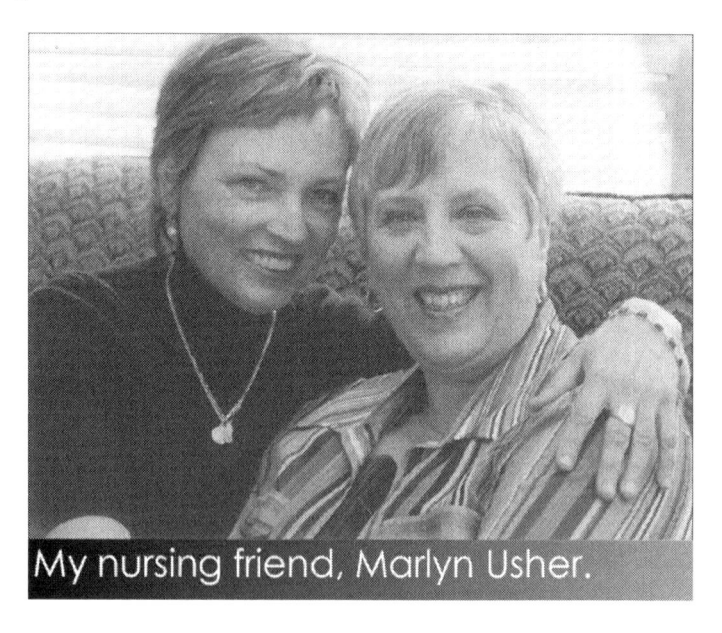

My nursing friend, Marlyn Usher.

I had received a two-day pass from the Brantford

Waking Up

General and Jim had brought me home. I couldn't understand this and thought Jim had brought me home for a few days before locking me away in the group home. My fantasies horrified me. I desperately didn't want to go to a group home shared by people, mostly older patients, restrained in wheelchairs, waiting to die.

I determined that I would avoid the dreaded group home at all costs. Being the resourceful farm-girl I am, I developed an escape plan and carefully packed my bags and strategically arranged them.

This was my brilliant plan. Jim's parents, the Whites, would want to come and see me once I had returned home and the time finally arrived to put my plan in action. Their car pulled into the long driveway and I heard the two dogs announce their arrival with a cacophony of barking.

They were bound to help me I reasoned. After all, hadn't Dr. White built a special railing on the staircase for me because my leg dragged? Just as they would go to leave, I would run out and get into their car. They lived near the hospital and I knew they would let me spend my last days with them if I threw myself upon their mercy. If my cancer got worse I would be near the Brantford General. Being compassionate people, I knew the Whites could not refuse me once I was in their car.

EMOTIONAL UPSET***

Your loved one may become easily upset, angry or frustrated. These are common behaviors after stroke. Behavior changes can be hard to deal with.

-Remind yourself that they do not have control of these behaviors.
-Think about how your loved one is feeling. Figure out the cause of the behavior.
-What was the trigger? Remove the trigger to prevent future incidents.

Waking Up

At that time, I could only go down the stairs like a toddler, sliding down each step on my bum, so I quietly did so. There I was, prepared, waiting in the hall, all set to run out with my bag, when I heard Jim call, "Crystal, your bath!". 'Damn,' I thought, 'Jim must know.'

I limped back upstairs, shut the bathroom door behind me and disrobed. I heard the car start up and the Whites leave down the long driveway. I sighed while the warm water and bubbles that Jim had prepared enveloped my body. "Somehow, he must have discovered what I was thinking."

However, I remember his care and I relaxed as he treated me like the new-born I was. I started to think maybe he wasn't such a bad guy after all and maybe someone else had stolen the ring. He had drawn me such a nice warm bath and provided me with clean-smelling, thick towels. As the mist rose over the top of the bath, I relaxed and luxuriated in the steam and the bubbles.

On returning to our bedroom, I finally figured out what was happening. While I was in the bath, Jim had taken the belongings out of my "escape" bag. He then began to lay out clothes from my drawers in little piles.

I knew it!, He was preparing to send me away to a group home. After I was dressed, Jim came to get me. I said, "No!", and refused to move. I grabbed the edges of the mattress tightly. I was just going to stay on that bed. No group home for me!

Jim was exasperated. In the end he had to call all three boys to "help" me into the truck. The three of them were all seasoned hockey players and Jim is no slouch himself, being a farmer. Together, they tore my hands off of the mattress and with all four of them controlling me, dragged me out of the door.

When Jim got me through the door, I grabbed onto the door handle and implored my sons, "Why won't you save

Waking Up

me?" Watching them ignoring my pleas just wasn't like them. My own sons. Why wouldn't they help me? Since I couldn't communicate with them, it was torture as Jim quietly forced me into the cab of the pickup and locked the seat belt.

I knew my sons were all in on the conspiracy but they couldn't be that cold. I was their mother! Looking back I can't decide whether it was a beautiful, or awful moment as we pulled out of the drive and left our farmhouse forever. I saw a tear in my son, James' eye. He did care after all.

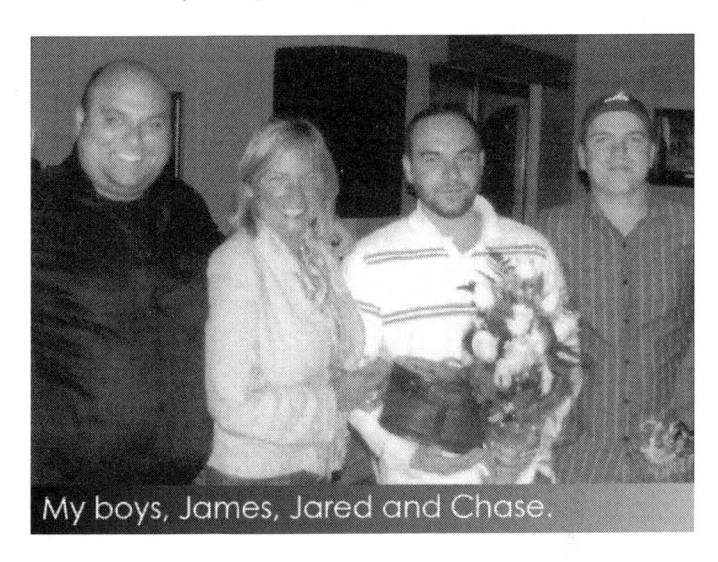

My boys, James, Jared and Chase.

It strikes me now that in my foggy recollection I was watching my boys grow into men before my eyes and it brought to mind nights of reading to them before bed-time. My favourite was that beautiful book by Robert Munsch, 'Love You Forever', where the mother sneaks in to her adult son's bedroom to hug him like a baby. My boys still cared for me!

As we pulled out of the long driveway, Jim struggled to hold me back. I was not going to go quietly. However, in the back of my mind, there was one thing about the

Waking Up

incident that didn't add up.

What truly puzzled me was that, despite all the screaming, fighting, pulling and yelling on the way out of the house to the truck, my breathing didn't seem to be a problem. I certainly wasn't winded, which was strange, since I was dying of lung cancer.

On the way to the dreaded group home in Brantford, I fought Jim periodically as he struggled to restrain me and keep the pickup on the road all the way to Brantford. Finally, in exhaustion and thinking of my boys, I gave in. Moving into the home would mean they wouldn't be burdened with me for the final days of my life.

It would be a blessing for them although it was a sad day for me as we entered Brantford on our way to the group home.

6 THE REHAB CONSPIRACY

To my surprise and joy, we pulled up to the Brantford General. My hospital. The hospital that I had worked thirty years in and a place where I had friends. It felt good to enter the lobby as I had done so many times before with its familiar Tim Hortons on one side and the volunteer gift shop on the other. As the doors of the elevator opened for us, I knew right away where I would be going – to Palliative Care on the 7th floor.

EMOTIONAL HELP***

Frustration at the inability to communicate can lead to paranoia, anger and depression. Family members may also feel strong emotions.

-Friends and other family members may be sources of support so talk with them
-Involve the stroke survivor in decision-making as much as possible
-Give them time to talk. Don't speak for him/her
-Use touch to communicate
-Acknowledge and verbalize the frustration your loved one feels

Waking Up

The elevator went up one floor and stopped. I was confused. Jim pushed the wheelchair out and I saw the sign, B2. At the Brantford General, B2 was the unit dedicated to caring for rehabilitation patients. I puzzled over it, then realized that there likely wasn't a bed available yet in Palliative Care and I would have to wait for one on the rehab floor. I had seen it happen before.

My friends at the hospital were still trying to help me understand and constantly dropping hints and giving me advice to the point of annoyance.

Every day the stroke nurse Anne Campbell, would visit and talk about stroke. I always liked Anne and it was nice to see her but I remember thinking, "Why waste your time with me? I'm dying of cancer."

Sometimes Jim came with her to push the pamphlets she gave him for me but I knew all about him. He was the one who had stolen my father's ring and he was just hanging out for the insurance settlement.

When Anne left and he stopped pressuring me to look at pamphlets, I changed my mind. Somehow he had

> **PRESCRIPTION FOR RECOVERY**
>
> The best way to get better after a stroke is to start stroke rehabilitation or "rehab".
>
> -You have the greatest chance of regaining your abilities during the first few months after a stroke.
>
> -It is important to start early and do a little every day.
>
> -You may recover the most in the first few weeks or months after your stroke.
>
> -You can keep getting better for years. It just may happen more slowly.

changed and he wasn't a villain. I smiled as he held my hand and murmured, "Go to sleep, go to sleep, go to sleeeeeppppp.....," and I drifted off to sleep.

My life became a constant round of tests and examinations. As the pain in my leg became more intense, I asked Dr Kagoma, a specialist at the Brantford General to test me for a deep vein thrombosis or DVT. This is a blood clot usually found in a deep vein in the body such as in the legs. I underwent an ultrasound exam and it came back clear.

When they wanted yet another chest x-ray at the Brantford General (I thought it was a chest exam but it was really a neurological scan) I refused to go. No more poking and prodding. Dr. Manning must have realized it was too much for me since he agreed to cancel it.

My sister, Jackie, bought me all new clothes. I remember a group of nurses gathered around the new shoes, complimenting me on them. As Jackie was cheerily hanging the rest of the clothes up in my closet and being positive and bouncy, I thought, "Why waste your money on someone who is dying?"

OCCUPATIONAL THERAPY*****

Occupational therapy, often called OT, is the use of treatments to develop, recover, or maintain the daily living and work skills of people with a physical, mental or developmental condition.

It was incredibly frustrating. I was a terminal case and yet the therapists were insisting that I get up onto a treadmill. After a few strides, I refused. I couldn't even tell them why I was saying, "No, No, No!" I felt trapped inside my damaged body.

Back to the ring conspiracy. The ring my father had given to me was the same one that I was sure Jim had stolen was very special to me. It was my dad's ring and now it had disappeared.

One day, my son James showed up with the ring. It turned out that when I arrived in Buffalo, my fingers were so swollen, the nurses in the Operating Room had to cut it off my finger. James had taken it to a jeweler in Burford and had them re-size it for my fingers.

It was the beginning of an understanding and slowly the cancer conspiracy in my world began to unravel.

Jim told me later that he took my frustration personally and felt that I was blaming him for my condition. I had no idea at the time. When I was released from the hospital two weeks later, I still didn't get it. I simply figured that I was going to last a little longer, thinking, "two weeks, two months, two years, who knows?"

Rehabilitation therapy made no sense to me and I remember being terrible at it. Karen, from home care tried to teach me about a microwave and she demonstrated opening cupboards for me.

Stepping onto the treadmill machine later, my frustration mounted, "I wasn't stupid, I just couldn't speak!" I got off of the treadmill in tears and made my way back to my room. Honestly, I was in a terrible mental state by the time I was able to begin speech therapy.

Here is how I saw it. I felt that the world had dealt me some cruel cards. Trapped inside myself, I couldn't speak one word, not one. It was slowly donning on me. That was the reality. I could barely understand others, let alone, speak.

The only glimmer of hope was a spontaneous recovery. I remember being shocked a few years before my stroke when I heard that my friend, Jim Cuddy, lead singer for the band Blue Rodeo, had lost his voice and was unable to speak, yet two weeks later his voice returned.

WAKING UP AT THE COTTAGE

Surprisingly, pictures made sense to me. Dr. White showed me how the bleeding aneurysm affected half of my brain.

> **DRAW A PICTURE*****
>
> Stroke survivors with communication challenges can work around it by writing or drawing. They might supplement verbal expression with gestures, picture communication book, or computer technology.

I saw how they cut my skull open to relieve the pressure and where they put the piece of bone for safekeeping. I was now beginning to understand this.

I had been introduced to Jan Roadhouse, a speech language pathologist at the Brantford General as a fellow care-giver at the Brantford General before my stroke. I connected with her immediately and admired her skills.

Our relationship progressed further as I got to know her better as an inpatient on the rehabilitation unit. I was pleased to know that this incredible woman would be treating me as an out-patient in her community rehabilitation program. Like my speech patterns, my writing was broken and difficult to understand. I was basically starting as a baby, waking up at square one.

I developed a deep bond with Jan as we worked with each other over the years. A very gentle soul, she never pushed or pressured me. She was always encouraging and gave me hope for recovery.

I looked forward to our sessions together and admired her dedication. Due to the hospital restrictions on therapy costs, she was only allowed to work part-time. Those who know Jan, however will attest to the fact that she always worked over-time for her patients.

She constantly seemed amazed at my sense of humour about my condition. One day she made me laugh with a suggestion that seemed ridiculous to me but strangely interesting. She said, "Crystal, you just have to write a book!". She thought my humour and my perspective, as a nurse who worked on a stroke floor prior to her stroke, would be unique.

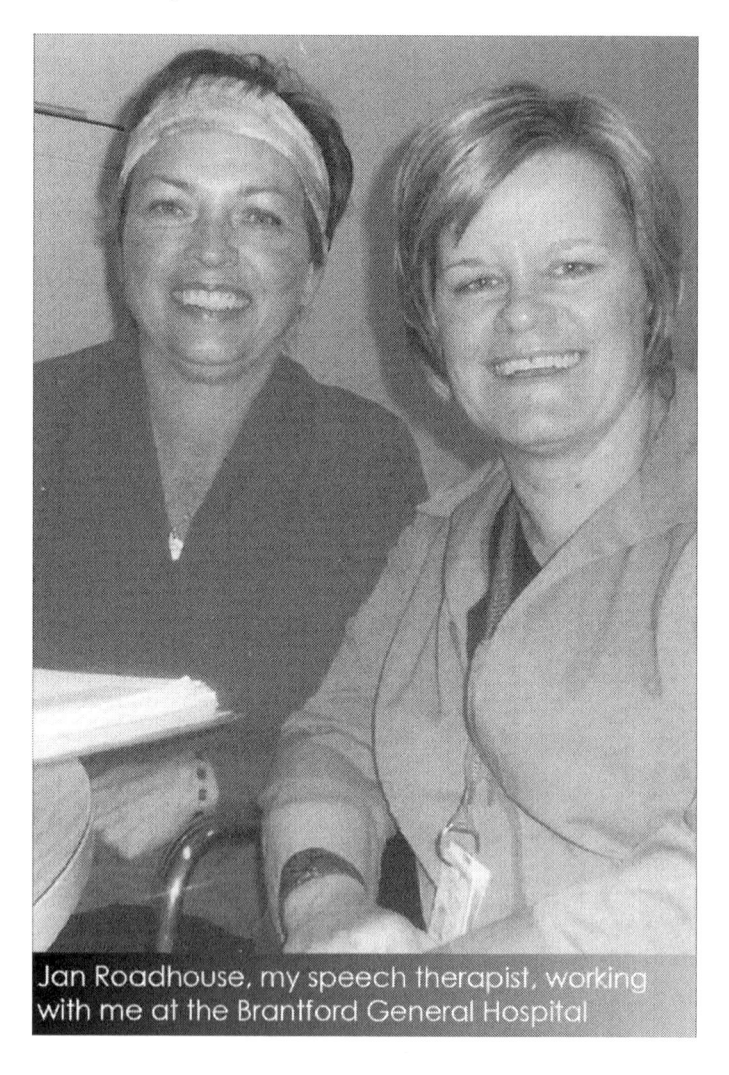

Jan Roadhouse, my speech therapist, working with me at the Brantford General Hospital

Waking Up

I was intrigued but when I thought about it realistically, I could barely spit out a word at a time. It just didn't seem possible. Well here it is many years later and I am glad to say, Jan's prediction came true.

During an initial session as an outpatient of Jan's, I scribbled down 'CA?'. Now any normal person might think that I was trying to write that as part of a web address or something. However, Jan, knowing the nursing abbreviations that are used in hospitals recognized it right away. "Do you have cancer?" There was a long pause..."That is something you will have to ask Dr. Manning about the next time you see him," she said.

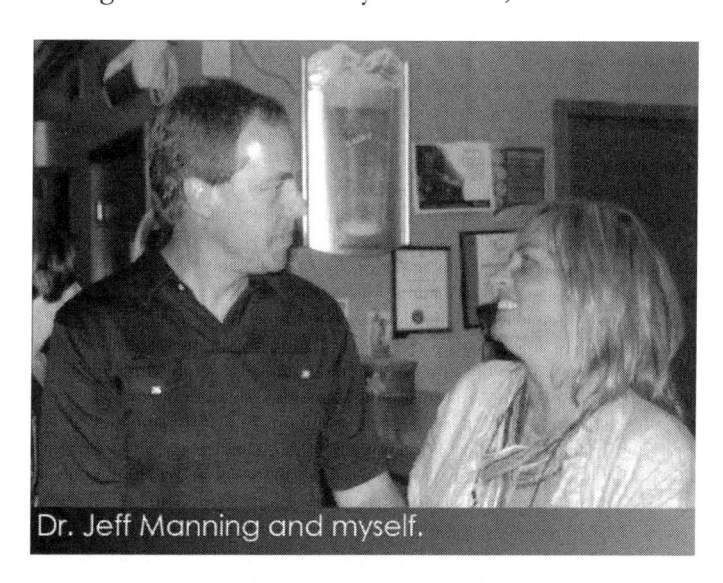

Dr. Jeff Manning and myself.

Jeff Manning was my family physician and I knew I could talk to him about anything and he would be truthful and educational. He is an excellent healer and I trust him implicitly.

One day I spied Dr. Manning in the hallway of the Brantford General Hospital, visiting his patients. I managed to make myself understood when I scribbled, "CA". He looked at me seriously and shook his head, making me understand, saying, "No Crystal, you are not dying of cancer."

Thank you Jeff. That day you successfully helped to put an end to the fog of my conspiracy theories.

Things started to fall together and the truth began to emerge. Later that night, looking in the mirror, I stuck my tongue out, and there it was, a definite pull to the right, a most obvious clinical sign. As a nurse, I recognized it right away as a sure sign of stroke.

WAKING UP - WITH A LITTLE HELP

In the early hours of the next morning, I had a very strange sensation. It was something I felt since waking up from the coma. There was something, or someone, waiting over my left shoulder. I knew it was a calming, healing presence that I sensed was watching over me.

For two years as my speech slowly improved it stayed by my side. One day I woke up and it was gone. "It's okay, I don't need you now," I said, "you can move on to another person who needs you." Waking up, I knew I was on my way to recovery.

7 BACK ON MY FEET

I had my final surgery in Hamilton where Dr. Rocco Devilliers did a "replacement bone flap."

He put the piece of my skull back which they had taken out in Buffalo and put in my abdomen for safe keeping. The surgery went well and it wasn't long before I was back up on my feet. For me, that was a real, measurable, milestone.

There was one final fantasy that I had been holding on to. I was sure that once I had the last operation and the piece of skull was back into its rightful place in my head, I would wake up and be talking, just like before.

I had a keen sense of disappointment when that did not happen. However, all the operations were finished and I could now

> **MEDICATION MAYHEM**
>
> "Stroke victims must be very careful about altering their medication routine. Some drugs such as those affecting the nervous system are quite powerful and any changes must be made in cooperation with your physician. Doing otherwise can cause severe problems such as withdrawal symptoms."
>
> Dr. Thorsteinn Gunnarson, Neurologist

seriously focus on re-learning how to speak.

A word to the wise, a little knowledge can be a dangerous thing. A month later, I was still on the same prescription medication as when I had left Buffalo. As a nurse I started to seriously question them, especially the pain medications and the anti-depressants. I was not in pain and I certainly wasn't mentally ill! So I just stopped taking them. Boy, was I wrong. I woke up in the middle of the night with half my face twitching madly and realized I had made a mistake.

When I next saw Dr. Manning, he explained to me, "Crystal, those are strong medications. You can't just stop them. You have to be weaned off them." When I questioned the anti-depressant, he said bluntly, "You have to take that. Without it your brain will not heal."

Privately, I wondered if the anti-depressants would have been more useful if I had been taking them before my stroke to help with the combined stresses of working while raising three boys.

For the longest time I called Dr. Manning by his first name, "Allan." I honestly could not understand why everyone else was calling him, "Jeff."

Although I had known the name he went by pre-stroke, I didn't know him by any other name. In my coma I remember being told by a spirit that "Allan" was his name. I was convinced he was Allen, yet I heard others calling him Jeff. I couldn't understand why and it was a source of great confusion with me. It became clear to me when I noticed a plaque in his office, saying, "Allan Jeffery Manning". So that was where Jeff had come from.

I was grateful at that moment that my speech hadn't come back fully and he couldn't know what I was calling him. Coincidentally, his father, whom I also knew when he was alive, had passed away just and he was named "Allan."

Pain was a constant companion in my long journey to recovery. Trudging up the endless driveway from the parking garage to the Rehabilitation Centre, every step seemed to be a torture.

I complained of the pain I was feeling and Jan paged Dr. Manning. When he arrived, the explanation he had for me was embarrassingly simple, amusing and complimentary. He teased me, "Crystal, you're feeling pain because you have lost so much weight that there is no padding on your bones anymore."

> **Pain Management******
>
> Stroke victims will feel pain. Pain management may include medications but other tips are:
> -stress management
> -relaxation therapy
> -keeping active
> -eating healthy
> -physiotherapy exercises

Sometimes we all need a little help understanding and accepting, even if we think we can do it all ourselves.

Although I desperately wanted my independence and nine months after my stroke, I felt capable, others were not so sure. It was time for Kelly, the neighbour girls, Maryanne and Teresa and I to go on our annual November cross-border shopping trip. Maryanne and Teresa helped fill in as my care-givers when Kim or Kelly were busy. Worried about my state, they considered cancelling it but I wanted to go. I had even learned a word for the event, "Rum."

We headed out to the States and while we perused the items, Kelly lost sight of me. In a panic, she called out my name loudly and searched through the store as if I were a child.

Hearing her looking for me, I had to laugh as it reminded me of shopping with my children when they were little. Although all this attention cramped my shopping style, I knew her heart was in the right place. From then on, I tried to stay in sight.

At that time Jim signed me up for a telephone alarm system. I had to wear a necklace with a button on it so if I was in trouble, I could call for help. I wasn't crazy about this "baby monitor" thing but we kept the subscription for the next couple of years.

MUSIC THERAPY*****

Music Therapy has been medically proven to be a valuable tool after a stroke. It can assist in areas of movement and muscle control, speech and communication, cognition, mood and motivation.

I was still upset emotionally and feeling pretty down. To cheer me up, Arlene and her husband Don arranged to get tickets to see my favourite musician, Jim Cuddy. He is a good friend of ours and I was looking forward to seeing Jim again.

Arriving at the Norfolk Fairground in Simcoe and entering the stadium, I realized that our seats were in the section closer to the back. As a good friend of Jim, I was used to getting seats closer to the stage.

My disappointment wasn't helping my emotional state and I was starting to feel pretty small and shrunk back into my seat. It wasn't a concert I was looking forward to. Looking back I know that my brain wasn't coping so well with all of the trauma we had been through together.

However, I am a firm believer that God gives you what you need to heal and it isn't all about surgeries and medications. Jim Cuddy had known that I was coming and he instinctively knew how to help me.

After the first set of songs, I heard my name from the stage, "This song is for my good friend Crystal." He began to sing, "Try," a particularly apt choice for aphasia patients.

Waking Up

After that magical moment I was transported into the familiar, beautiful world of Jim's music. Like the groupie I am, I went to the front of the stage and threw him a kiss. Thank you Jim Cuddy for helping bring me through the rough times and heal me with music.

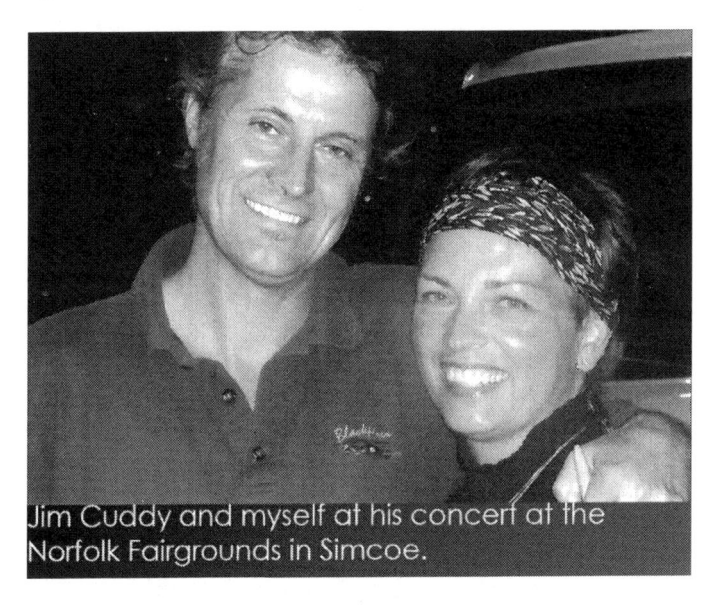

Jim Cuddy and myself at his concert at the Norfolk Fairgrounds in Simcoe.

CHORUS TO "TRY" BY JIM CUDDY
Oh you got to try, try, try.
Ah don't you know you've got to try, try, try.
Oooh Oh baby you try, oh.

GOOD ADVICE*****

Speakeasy is a conversational practice group in Cleveland, Ohio. Among their tips for communicating with speech and language limitations in social settings is:
• Try, try, try to get your point across no matter what anybody says or thinks.

8 GROWING UP - AGAIN

I was floating again, but this time, it wasn't heavenly. The pain coursed through my body. I saw fire and the vision of fire seemed all too real. The thought crept into my mind, "Is this the Devil?"

I squirmed in bed but it wasn't something I could escape. For some strange reason, I was sure it was all related to that first cigarette that I had when I was younger. Why did I have to do that?

As I struggled in pain, my last thought was instructional - "This is not the right place for me!" I forced myself to awaken. I woke up to life. I determined right then and there that there was no way I was going to hell. Since I wouldn't call myself religious in any way, my visit to hell was frightening.

My dad was an Anglican, my mother was Greek Orthodox and the local Church is a United Church so I thank my lucky stars that I had plenty of Christian choices. Not long after I came home, my minister called and asked if he could speak with me. I refused to see him. I told him, "I'm not ready to die yet!" I really wasn't ready to go to either heaven or hell.

Surprisingly to some, I felt my surroundings were like a living funeral. At first the house was constantly filled with flowers making it smell and look like a funeral home. To top it all off, for two solid years, our mailbox was full of condolences and get well cards, constantly reminding me of a funeral. It wasn't such a bad thing after all. It was gratifying to be see so much support from family and friends. Why do we have to wait for a funeral? It doesn't do us much good then. I much prefer the way it happened to me.

NO PEN, NO PAPER!

Speech Therapy is so important to me. I am not one for sign language. My brain doesn't work that way. I have to talk and I set about re-learning my words with a passion. Although not speaking yet, I was determined to be understood.

I remember my first meeting with Jan. It was just after I had my operation to replace the piece of skull in my forehead. I was frustrated because I had expected to speak after that and it just didn't happen.

Showing her my pen and a stack of papers, I then swept them off her table and onto the floor. I think Jan got the message pretty quickly. Through all of my motioning and pantomiming she understood very clearly that I wanted to relearn speech and not rely on a pen and paper to

> **SPEECH THERAPY**
>
> Speech-language pathologists (SLPs), also called speech and language therapists, or speech therapists, specialize in the evaluation and treatment of communication disorders and swallowing disorders.

communicate.

Like any great teacher with years of experience, Jan was a gold mine and I couldn't get enough of her.

I love Jan and I am sure she wouldn't mind me saying this, but it is partly because of her big mouth! Seriously. I even had Kim film her as she demonstrated how the mouth works for common words. The video was a brilliant idea that Kim had and I relied on the technique for years.

Sitting in Jan's windowless office on the third floor of "D" wing there was a momentous occasion when I spoke my first word. It was "Mom". It took me so long before I could do it. It was a whole week, full-time, to learn that one.

Watching intently how Jan's mouth worked on the video, I resolutely played it back over and over. I think "Mom" was my first word because, as a mother myself, I empathized with my mother, having children to care for and one who now needed special caring for. When we are young, we don't have any idea how tough it is to raise us, the children. Now that I had my own, I could see all that my mother had done for us and continues to do for us now that she is "79ish".

I had also mastered the word, "hi,". I nervously prepared to greet my mother with the two words. She seemed pleased but, like most parents, wanted more out of me. She declared, "Good. Now you can learn 'hello'."

My mother, Jennie.

Waking Up

I did go on to learn 'hello', but saying "Mom," was the best feeling and filled me with hope. I said to myself, "I am healing my brain!" It was a small but important victory.

In some ways re-learning words could become fun and I liked how they came more naturally as I practiced. I liked working on my brother-in-law's name Dave Thomson and worked on the sound "D". For the longest time, I took pleasure in saying his name which had become "Da...Da...Da...Dave," which made him laugh.

The next triumph was tackling that all important Canadian icon, Tim Hortons. Although ordering coffee was a struggle, both for the girl serving me and myself, I struggled on with great tenacity and was finally rewarded with a hot cup of coffee. I don't humiliate easily!

I took my lessons seriously, still not able to work or drive, trapped in Hatchley, but it didn't matter to me. I knew my real job was re-learning to speak. Due to my circumstances, I felt like a prisoner and each new word I learned represented freedom.

I needed to learn how the sound "G" sounded like bullfrogs and how "H" was like the sound of my breathing as I gave birth, a very personal approach to sound.

Frustrated at not being able to make a "B" or a "D" sound, I was amazed as Jan gently put my hand on her larynx to match the vibration. It worked! Small successes built up.

I remember noting how different my voice sounded just after my stroke. Gradually, over the months it began to return to normal and the sound of my voice changing back was a good sign of healing as I progressed in my recovery.

There is a strategy of combining words that I found to be very effective. I worked for weeks on the name of my dog Izzy - (Is he?). My friend is a pilot but I simply could not say the word no matter how hard I tried. Jan said to me, "Why don't you combine two words you know already, 'pie' and 'lot.'" It worked and I could say, "Pie-lot". That strategy also worked for my favourite coffee. The letter, "d" and a baby cow became "d'calf."

However, there are some things that are beyond speech rehabilitation and I still call them a him, or him a her or vice versa. They/him/her who know about my condition don't seem to mind.

> **CONVERSATION AIDS*****
> • Establish a topic first
> • Ask yes/no questions
> • Paraphrase during conversations
> • Try different lengths and complexity of conversations
> • Use gestures to emphasize important points

Throughout my long rehabilitation, an incident one morning stuck in my mind and drove me to greater efforts.

I was visiting my neighbour, Ruth and holding a little bundle of girl in my arms, her granddaughter, Grace. She was so adorable and comfortable. I thought of my family, looked at Ruth and told myself determinedly, "I will speak!"

You see, at that time we lived on a farm in a rural area, quite distant from others, with only a few neighbours. I knew there would be grand-children. Yet, I understood that I would never be able to be with them by myself. How could I if I couldn't call 911? I didn't even know how to say it! It just wouldn't be safe for anyone concerned.

That is why one of my first sentences was "Call 911". That is an issue most people are not confronted with. What words are important to learn first?" At home I applied myself to the task. As I practiced my alphabet out loud, it was a struggle to remember what came after the letter "C". The dictionary became a constant companion.

It has been an interesting journey through my brain, learning how to reconnect thoughts after a stroke. Early in my recovery, I found that whispering helped me to practice.

It wasn't as difficult as speaking aloud and helped me to continue longer. During a long day alone at our house in Hatchley, I was looking at our cat and trying to say her name to get her to come. I surprised myself by speaking in a deep, sexy voice, "Dusteee". She came up to me and glided her body across my leg. It was easier than speaking normally!

Mind you, I don't speak like this all the time, or my male friends might get the wrong idea, but when I have trouble getting out a word, it sometimes helps.

HINT, DON'T CORRECT

Facilitate, rather than correct. If it is a wrong word or gesture, avoid correcting them. Give a hint instead.
-If you think they are trying to say "purse", you could face them and say "puh"
-Try writing down what they are trying to say, as reading it may help.
-Give them a pen and paper, a calendar or newspaper to help them get their message out in a different way.
-Making the hand movement for something (such as bringing the hand to the mouth to indicate "eat") might help them to get the word out.

I know that some stroke survivors can't speak a word, yet they can sing whole songs. The brain is an amazing organ. At one point I was referred to a sign language instructor but it didn't make much sense to me. Even if I learned sign language, the people I most wanted to communicate with wouldn't know it. I wanted to be able to speak to them.

Three days a week for two years Kim, Kelly and I faithfully made our way to Jan's office at the Brantford General. What great women I am privileged to know.

MY RECORDING SESSION

One day, while working with Jan in her office, she asked me what songs I knew. Surprised, I told her that I didn't know any songs. She looked at me coyly and said, "Come on Crystal, everyone knows a song." I thought about it and wrote down, "Happy Birthday."

That began a long period of re-learning the words to the song. Kim and Jan would laugh every time we would practice the song but before long I realized that I was going to be able to learn the song and began planning for my recording session. Kim later confessed to me that it was very painful for her but she would try to cheer me up each time.

In the coming month, there were three friends of mine who would be celebrating their birthdays, Mrs. White, my friend Paul and Jim Cuddy.

I practiced every day and finally the big day came. I knew the words to the entire song and had picked up three of those greeting cards that you can record a message on. I sang the song into each, autographed them and sent them away.

At her cottage, when Mrs. White revealed the card she had received from me she opened it up. As it began to play, the sound of my voice coming from her card brought my mother-in-law to tears. Later, when she called me up to thank me she said that, "hearing you sing was the best birthday present of my life!"

9 RECOVERY

When I decided to get serious about writing this book, a very dear friend, Scott, offered me his cottage to stay at. It overlooked the cliffs of Lake Erie and I just loved it. A cozy little house perched at the edge with a view of Long Point in the distance. I brought some light reading for the summer. I know it is just baby steps, but for me it was huge. I did get through the first four pages of the primary book, "Bear's Vacation", a small but important victory.

Lately I have had to deal with the passing of both Mrs. White and Dr. White who were treasured parts of my life. It gave me great pleasure to be there when Dr. White was able to come to my son's wedding.

Once he called me at his cottage in Haliburton and challenged me. I remember it as a blessing in disguise. Mel, my son's wife, answered the phone for me. Dr. White insisted that I talk to him directly, so I got on the phone.

Dr. White said, "I don't

> **PHONE TIPS**
>
> When talking on the phone with a new person, it is helpful to learn the phrase, "I'm a stroke survivor...can you understand me?"

want Mel, only you!" He proceeded to give me instructions on how to operate the digital camera that he had given me earlier. Despite his best efforts, I had to interrupt him to say, "Dad, I am not able to understand, it is too much for me."

I hated to disappoint him, but it was a good lesson.

What I learned was this; sometimes even though I give it my best effort, it is okay to recognize my limits. It is always a struggle and you will rarely get it right the first time. We all need understanding and it might help for others to look at it from our viewpoint and practice patience with stroke victims.

People with Aphasia all agree that people speak too fast to understand. "Repeat" is becoming my favourite word and I use it anytime I need to.

I love to make pies and found it was to be a major part of my therapy. I enjoyed re-learning how to do this. I made pies for dinner, pies for gifts, pies for neighbours, pies for funerals, pies for weddings.

> **RESTAURANT TIPS**
>
> If waiters/waitresses speak too fast when you go out to dinner, let them know you are a stroke survivor and ask them to slow down.

I was proud of myself for having made all 30 pies for my niece, Lyndsay's wedding at her family's cottage in Muskoka. I know that Jim and Kelly were hard-pressed to keep up with my constant demand for new fruit, flour and sugar but this was something that I could do for others. Little did I know, but this was occupational therapy in action.

Something that surprised Jim about my condition were the constant trips he had to make for groceries. In addition to the pie ingredients, for some reason, during this stage in my recovery, I had serious food cravings, especially for fish and watermelon. It was exactly like being pregnant again!

There I was trapped in Hatchley without a license so I did what made me comfortable and made my pies (and good ones at that). Although it was an art to be re-learned, it was something that didn't change with my stroke. It just took me a while to remember how to create a great pie and it was great therapy to do so.

That must have been quite a sight. Me in my Hatchley kitchen, covered in flour, trying to remember recipes, dragging my leg around and dancing to the music of Jim Cuddy and Blue Rodeo. But who cares about how you look? It is how the pies taste! I am sure that if you visit me at my house today in Brantford, everyone will vouch that I am still the undisputed and reigning, "Kitchen Queen", something I am quite proud of.

And the result of my pride was, one fall morning I ran afoul of my mother-in-law, whom I adored. I came downstairs to find her washing the kitchen floor. Keep in mind that my driving license had been rescinded and I was virtually trapped in the farmhouse. A tone of desperation had crept into my imprisonment.

Seeing her washing my floor on her hands and knees was just too much for me to bear. I grabbed the cloth and even though my right leg dragged around a bit, I was determined to clean my own kitchen floor. I needed to be independent. To this day, I have regretted hurting her feelings, but I feel she understood since she just quietly stepped back and watched me as I struggled on my hands and knees also.

Another curious effect of stroke was my changing vision. Sitting down to eat with my family, I noticed that I couldn't tell what was on my plate. It was all blurry. I also noticed that my field of vision narrowed in the early days and gradually came back over the next year.

That meant a trip to the optometrist and a new pair of

glasses. Wearing them one evening at dinner, my son, Jared, not used to seeing me with them on, joked with me, "Come on mom, you don't need glasses, you're not blind."

I guess his words worked on my sense of vanity because I never wear my glasses to dinner any more. Luckily, my vision has returned and I can now see what is on my plate.

I did have some fun with Dr. Manning when he was giving me a checkup. I pretended not to understand what he was saying to me and each time he asked me, I stepped closer like I couldn't see him. He must have thought my vision was becoming slightly blurry until I leaned forward as I got him in range and gave him a big fat kiss on the lips. Jim knowing how I am, just sighed loudly from his seat.

> **VISION LOSS**
>
> Vision loss is an area that a person cannot see. A stroke occuring in the left hemisphere can affect the right visual field of each eye, while right hemisphere stroke can impair the left visual field of each eye.
>
> - **Hemianopia** means blindness in one half of the visual field. Eight to ten percent of stroke survivors have it.
> - **Quadrantanopia** means blindness in a quarter of the visual field.
> - **Scotoma** refers to an island-like area of blindness.
> - **Tunnel vision** means peripheral vision is lost.

I struggled to communicate and took copious notes for my book. It was excellent therapy and very healing. Although I thought the notes were for my book when I gave them to Peter, I was shocked when he didn't want to use them. To be fair, looking over them later, I couldn't really understand them either. However, for my recovery it was, and still is, an important part of my rehab.

As I recovered, the connections in my mind began to

grow. I remember being in the General Store in Norwich and hearing the phrase, "yeah, yeah, yeah." It made me laugh and I called my sister, Jackie to tell her about it. She mentioned that the movie, "Divine secrets of the Ya-Ya Sisterhood had just come out so I would probably be hearing more of it." Yeah, Yeah, Yeah is a very useful and easy phrase for me.

Eventually I learned to use my camera and it became my security blanket throughout that time. I also found solace in taking long walks with our dogs through the fields on the farm. At times, our cat, Dusty, would tag along. Somehow taking pictures helped me with my memory. Now that I am talking better I leave my camera at home.

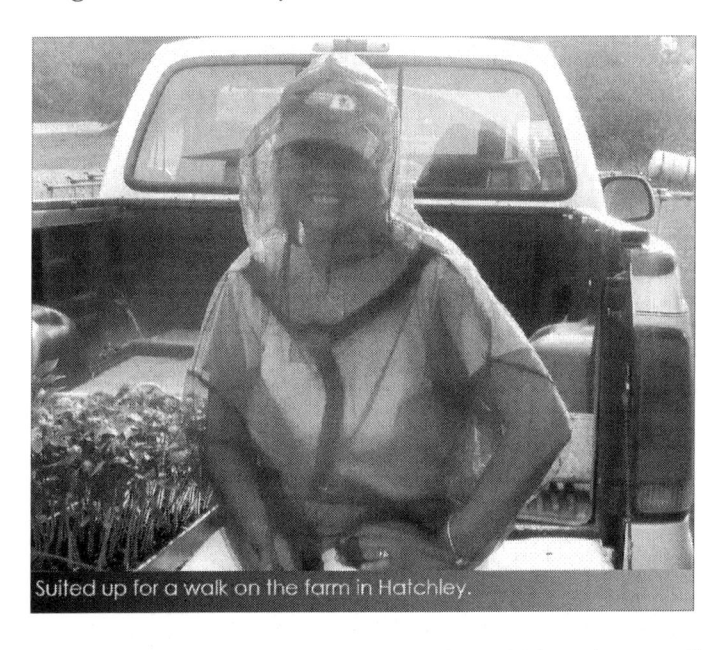

Suited up for a walk on the farm in Hatchley.

At first Jim worried about my safety during these walks and he wanted to come along. However, I took these walks to calm my mind and get away from my frustration with communication. When Jim tried to talk with me, I would get upset with him. We finally settled on a compromise. I made him walk ahead of me about 50 yards. I felt bad for him but I had good reason to insist as I needed the quiet time to heal. Later I changed my walking pattern to always be visible from our house.

On these long walks I would sometimes see hopeful signs. Once, as I walked through the forest, I looked up and saw something stuck in the crook of a tree. When I got closer, I saw that it was a bible. I picked it up, opened it and discovered it was from a church in Detroit. It was a wonderful find and made me feel as if I was being watched over.

On another excursion, I thought of my Grandma Jefferies. She was always one to look for four-leaf clovers. Although rare she often found them and proclaimed her luck loudly. I looked down at my feet and I was standing in a field of clover. Within a minute I had found four four-leaf clovers. I knew she was watching over me.

Learning numbers was one of the hardest parts of my recovery and, by far, the hardest was "ten". I finally got it walking the fields of Hatchley. The fields I was walking through were planted with ginseng and the posts for each row had a number displayed. As I walked past them, I would repeat the number.

Looking around at the beautiful, quiet and peaceful surroundings I began to feel strangely lucky. Working so hard to be a good nurse and raise a family, I had never been able to take the time to enjoy nature and see the seasons change on our farm. I wouldn't have had that experience if I hadn't had my stroke.

It is probably a good thing that our place in Hatchley was located in such a remote rural area since the sight of a woman in a ginseng field walking back and forth talking to herself might have been a little disturbing to the neighbours.

10 YOU SPEAK REALLY GOOD ENGLISH

It can be hard work trying to communicate and it can be very tiring for people with aphasia to be in social settings for any length of time. Within a large group of people there is a lot going on and it is difficult for those with aphasia to focus. Kim has noticed this process in me. It can be very overwhelming. I arrive in great spirits but as the night wears on, I eventually close-in on myself and retreat by the end of the party. I am better at social gatherings now, but they still tire me.

That May I had just been released from the Brantford General. Kelly and my friends were going to Port Dover for some perch and drinks. This was something we had done before and it always involved some good times. Although I wasn't feeling that great, I asked if I could go with them.

After the requisite drinks and food, we hit the stores to do some shopping. I managed to make it through the first few and then I hit a wall and began fading. It was all too much, the people, the talking, the clothes...following the fourth store, Kelly found me crying at the back of the store and realized I had overdone it. They cut the trip short and took me home. I still had fun but, like a toddler, I needed my morning and afternoon naps.

When I was first recovering from my stroke, I was astonished at how easily I would end up in tears. At first it was three or four times a day. Now this had gone down to once or twice a week.

It started to make sense when I was crying in front of my Uncle Carl. He hugged me and told me that it reminded me of my Aunt Olga. She had suffered with Multiple Sclerosis and she often cried as it was one of the symptoms of her disease. I realized that like her, crying was a symptom of my recovery from stroke and it would happen more often when I was frustrated or tired.

> **Consistent Crying**
>
> Damage to certain parts of the brain can reduce emotional control and increase tearfulness. Stroke patients can begin crying due to depression or even when happy. Usually it stems from the frustration of not being able to communicate.
> -It helps to stay quietly for a few moments and then try to divert their attention with a gentle pat or reassuring hug.

My sister, Kim asked me to go with her for the week when she went to a conference in Calgary. I leapt at the chance. After a long flight, we went into a coffee shop where I ordered a coffee. A Chinese girl overheard my stilted conversation. She said to me, "You speak very good English," asking me if I was English, French or Swedish. I thought of correcting her but I was really tired, so I gave in and nodded my head at, "Swedish". In a way it was fun to imagine that I could speak again, just not in English. I had that feeling of acceptance again.

I met an interesting man while I was there. I was asking

for decaf coffee and wasn't getting my point across. I got a tea instead, so I went into the kitchen to let them know. After I had successfully explained myself to the waitress, I went back to my table with the decaf. A man sitting at a table opposite the kitchen asked me if I was a stroke patient. I told him, "Yes."

He then told me that his name was Blair and he was a victim of stroke as well. Once he mentioned it, I knew right away. Since he was young, not many people would see past that. He got his own coffee and joined me. In our conversation, he mentioned that his first words were, "Why Me?"

This was a question I too had struggled with. When I started to feel like I was the unlucky one, I thought of all the other people worse off than me. Maybe for some reason, I was chosen to have a stroke because I had the strength to handle it.

I told Blair that I was just grateful it happened to me and not to other members of my family. He nodded and agreed that we should be grateful, telling me that by surviving his stroke he went on to own the restaurant we were sitting in. Blair invited me to come back for breakfast the next day. Never one to turn down a free meal, I did and we had another good conversation.

They talk a lot about stroke survivor groups. That didn't work so well for me always being the youngest person there. Every stroke is the same as a person's thumbprint and everyone is different. I actually like meeting stroke victims in other settings.

At that time, my recovery began to get media attention. Peter Muir, the author of this book, had featured my story in Vim and Vigour Magazine. One thing led to another and Brian Thompson, a photographer from the Brantford Expositor, a local newspaper, came out to the farm, took some pictures of me and Gary Chalk wrote a feature article in Vibrant Magazine about me.

Reading the articles and becoming interested in my story, a couple, Walter and Dianne McTaggart called Jan Roadhouse to ask if she would approach me about meeting with their son, Murray, who was recovering from a stroke.

I ended up meeting Murray and his wife Julie at the McTaggart's house in Brantford. Despite our strokes being different types, Murray and I had a lot to compare. We were both relatively young when we had our strokes, with his happening when he was 42. We had both lost our speech and struggled to re-learn it.

At that point in my recovery, I told him that his speech was better than mine. I couldn't help but empathize with him. Murray went from being an accomplished swimming athlete to just managing being ambulatory and moving around. It is amazing how stroke affects people. Murray swims really well.

I get it, I went from an active nurse and mother to re-learning pretty well everything. Stroke and recovery from it can be a difficult process and sometimes it helps to talk about similar experiences. Sometimes it doesn't. Wally and Dianne have remained my friends to this day.

In the first year of my recovery, I was just learning to talk. In the second year I was talking but not that well. By the beginning of the fourth year I wanted to improve my practice but was only allowed so much rehabilitation time with Jan. I was frustrated because I could see results and knew if I had additional sessions it could help me.

Jim was able to get me coverage to work with a private Speech Language Pathologist, Amy O'Connell who works for Lear Communication in Ancaster. When I first met with her she picked up that numbers were a major problem for me. I had trouble with counting as I would constantly forget what number came after the other. Remembering lists such as the numbers that come after ten or what letters came after C continually stumped me. I could eventually remember them but putting that into words that people could understand was a challenge.

Word association helped in my quest. For example, my new cell phone number was something I struggled with so I associated the beginning number set, 226, with my son Chase' age at the time - 22 and the month he was born in -6 to remind me of it. I did the same with the rest of the numbers and eventually was able to remember my cell number.

People can be puzzled by the activities of stroke patients. I remember one friend caught me staring intently at her mouth. She paused, looked at me and leaned over saying, "Do I have something in my teeth?" I replied, "No, I'm just looking at your throat." I really wanted to see how she was shaping her words and using her vocal cords.

Another time I was asked to take a picture of a group of friends. I was fascinated by a five year old child, Koehen saying the word, "cheese," with his mouth being so expressive. I'm not sure what he thought of the woman with the camera who kept making him repeat "cheese," but I am forever grateful to that little person for teaching me that. I like cheese.

Children are like little therapists for me. My friend Michelle's young daughter, Eliza, was forever trying to teach me to pronounce words. She kept telling me that, "when you have trouble with a word, just sound it out." She would then proceed to sound out the word for me... "fa, fa, fa, fall." How cute is that?

MY BUCKET LIST

At that point in my recovery, I started wanting to give back and started a list. You know that movie with Jack Nicholson and Morgan Freeman? They meet in a hospital after finding out both of them have terminal cancer. The movie is about them completing their "bucket list", the things you want to do before you kick the bucket. Well after my near-death experience that gave me a taste of my own mortality, I began to develop a bucket list as well.

You are reading one of the items on my list. I hope you are finding it useful. Another was letting those who had a big impact on my life know how important they were to me. I had always wondered what had happened to my teacher in Grade four and six, Ted Wilson.

Every time I would think about my old public school days I thought I should try to find out where he was. So one day I walked into the school and enquired about him.

They told me that he had retired so I left them my number to see if he wished to get together. I was thrilled to hear his voice when he called and we arranged to meet at the East Side Mario's restaurant beside the local Wal-Mart store. Or so I thought I had.

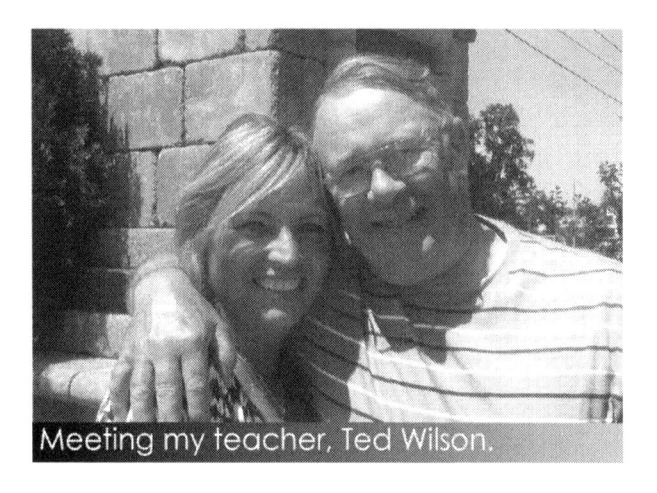

Meeting my teacher, Ted Wilson.

I arrived on time and sat down, nervously waiting to meet someone I hadn't seen in over forty years. The appointed time came and went. I started to sweat. Where was he? I got up and scanned the restaurant. I stood at the door looking for anyone who might look like him. Luckily my nursing friend, Sandy and her husband walked in. She greeted me. Then, seeing the state I was in, asked me if

Waking Up

anything was wrong.

I told her about meeting Ted and how it was important to me. Like most of my "guardian angels," she jumped in right away. Looking up his number on her phone, she called him and he answered. It turned out he thought we were meeting at the front door of the Wal-Mart store. After I didn't show up he returned home but offered to come back and see me.

By this time, all the emotion had worn me out and I was finding it a grueling experience to try and communicate. When he showed up we talked for about ten minutes, but I was fading fast so I arranged to meet him at another time. I did so with another school-mate, Allen, and it was great to talk with them both. I felt good that I let him know how important a teacher he was in my life and I could strike that one off my "bucket list."

My next stop was to the care team in Buffalo who saved my life. That seemed like a good moment to honour since my time there was barely a memory, yet that was where I was brought back to the living.

I planned a visit to the small group of physicians who were part of the team who put me back together. Most surgeons don't see their patients after they recover so this might be special for them.

I was proud of my progress and brought with me a case of Wayne Gretzky estate wine and Ferrero chocolates. The gifts represented some important stages in my recovery. My rehabilitation was tied into the Brantford General Hospital and Wayne Gretzky had grown up in Brantford. The Ferrero chocolates were given to me by the Foundation for my volunteer work, which I was proud of as well.

When the group of physicians saw me, they were amazed at the fact that I was visiting again and bearing gifts.

I didn't really feel confident speaking in front of them so I grabbed a pad to communicate. Dr. Levy gently put the pad down, looked me in the eyes and asked me if I could speak. When I nodded, he said, "Then talk to me." I thought about it and then told them that I knew three words, "Beer, rum, wine!" Laughing, he responded with, "At that rate, you will be speaking in three years."

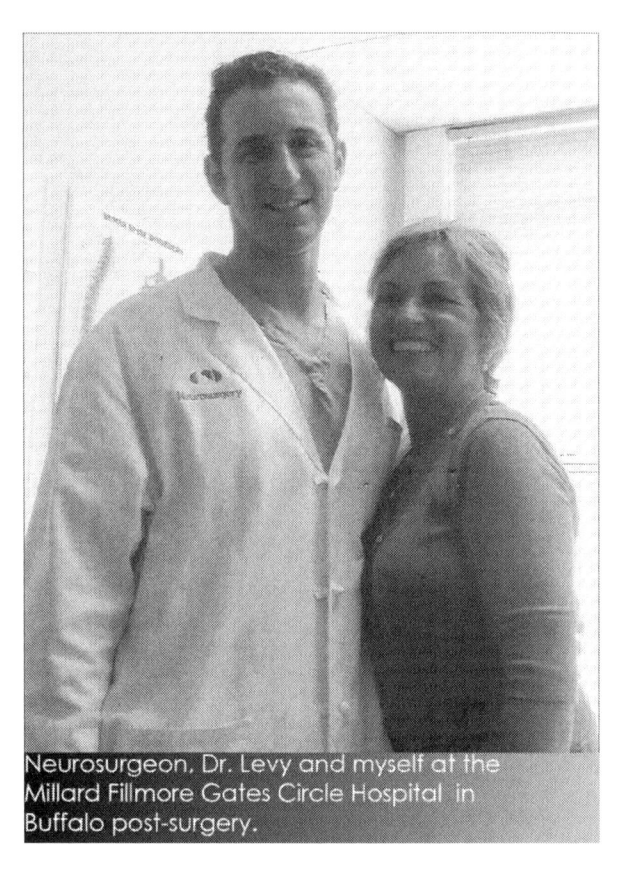

Neurosurgeon, Dr. Levy and myself at the Millard Fillmore Gates Circle Hospital in Buffalo post-surgery.

11 INDEPENDENCE/DEPENDENCE

At the tender age of five years old I learned a valuable lesson about independence. Living in a rural area, I had to take the school bus almost everywhere. Early in my school bus-taking days my mother put me on the bus in the morning for my very first swimming lesson. I felt like a grown-up, very independent and did fine getting there.

On the school bus coming home, I saw some of the kids getting off at a stop. I followed them and suddenly, there I was, alone with the other kids having been picked up by their parents. After frantic calls to the Police and searching the roads, my mother found me walking home. Fortunately I survived that incident. It taught me to never, ever follow others and think for myself.

The most important key to any successful stroke recovery is a solid support system. People who are willing to help you get back on your feet. I have so many people to thank that the list is practically endless, but at that time, my sister Kim, bless her, basically put her own life on hold for two years to devote driving me to my rehab appointments.

It became "Crystal" clear to me in one moment. I remember experiencing the moment of realization when

Kim was helping me to the bathroom. As we stood up and worked our way to the bathroom I became aware that I was literally and figuratively leaning on her. It just wasn't right. I'm the big sister and my little sister should be leaning on me, not me on her. That moment in the hallway pretty much sums up the independence dilemma stroke survivors have to cope with. We have a great need to get as independent as we can, but sometimes we have to grow into it and depend on others for a little while.

In our family, I have a few nicknames such as "Sister Superior," or the "Queen Bee," related to my take charge personality at all the family functions. It was a shock to all when the stroke changed that. But now that I needed their help, it was to come with much love by the armful.

And then there are those extended sisters. My neighbour Kelly was truly wonderful and in the beginning stages of my recovery stopped by every other day to see how I was getting along and take me grocery shopping.

She might have regretted it, when, at the supermarket I strolled up to a clerk to talk to him. Did I mention that shyness is not one of my problems? At that time I was still talking nonsense words, things like "norscum" or "nester".

Kelly was astonished at my behaviour and jumped in to help me. Since she didn't want to offend me she would try to translate but didn't tell him that I had a stroke...until I turned away and she whispered to him, "stroke." Letting people know you have a stroke is a good idea. You see, in my case, people can't see my condition because my face is hiding my brain injury.

Although Kelly is generally supportive of my speech vocabulary, there is one phrase she wished that I had never learned. Every time we went out, I didn't want to go to just one store. After all, jewelry is at a different store than clothes and you can't just get your groceries from one market. I am also a bargain-hunter, so whenever we got back in the car, I would pipe up, "just one more," and we would head off to the next stop...and the next stop...and the next etc.

My husband, Jim was incredibly patient but I know that he was happy when he could go golfing again.

There are also those who have no idea how they have helped my recovery. During the difficult days of my recovery, when I was stuck at home, all I could do was make pies, but I relished the music of Blue Rodeo and Jim Cuddy. They have no idea how they contributed to my recovery.

You may have heard of the famous movie where an odd group of gunslingers stand up for poor Mexican villagers, "The Magnificent Seven?". Well, I am part of my very own "Magnificent Seven." The "wild nurses' weekends" did create a bond amongst some amazing people, so when I had my stroke, a group of them got together to organize a support system for my care.

These people, Alana Stewart, Fran Cass, Judy Sayles, Sandra Byrne, Vickie Rutherford and Marg Maker were my life-savers. One of them would drop by every other day to help cook, clean or do whatever needed to be done and their support has been invaluable. In case you counted, there are only six in the Magnificent Seven. The seventh is me.

They also took me completely by surprise one night. Jim and I had decided to go out to dinner so I got ready to go order some fast food, a favourite and comfortable outing that you don't have to get dressed up for. When he pulled up to the Burford Golf and Country Club, I wanted to know why. He answered, "Well, I said I would take you out to dinner. Come on in." I wasn't dressed for it and this wasn't exactly my idea of where we should have dinner, so I simply refused to get out of the car. Jim said, "Okay, okay, I'll take you somewhere else. I just want you to come in first. I have a friend who wants to meet you."

Waking Up

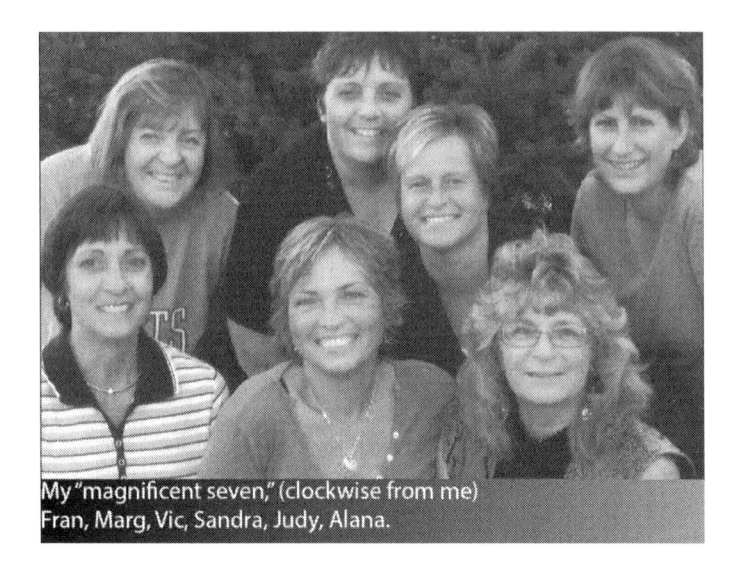

My "magnificent seven," (clockwise from me)
Fran, Marg, Vic, Sandra, Judy, Alana.

Reluctantly entering the darkened golf club, the lights came on and there was a loud chorus of, "Surprise!" The "Magnificent Seven" had organized a surprise "not-retirement" party and they had invited almost everyone they could think of. I saw friends from the hospital, family members and people I hadn't seen in thirty years.

The band that was playing for us that night, was "Doctor, Doctor" a great (and danceable) band composed of hospital staff I had worked with, all good friends of mine. They were a very popular band since releasing a video on YouTube that Peter Muir directed. It went viral and had over 65,00 views.

Best of all, my sister, Jackie, who I thought was in LA, had flown in to surprise me. It really worked. One of the band members and my good friend, Dr. Derek Dabreo, honoured me with a speech. He spoke of his admiration for my nursing skills, my compassion and my patience. He said that the night's recognition by my peers was all part of being an amazing nurse. It made the occasion into a very special evening for me and was great cause for celebration.

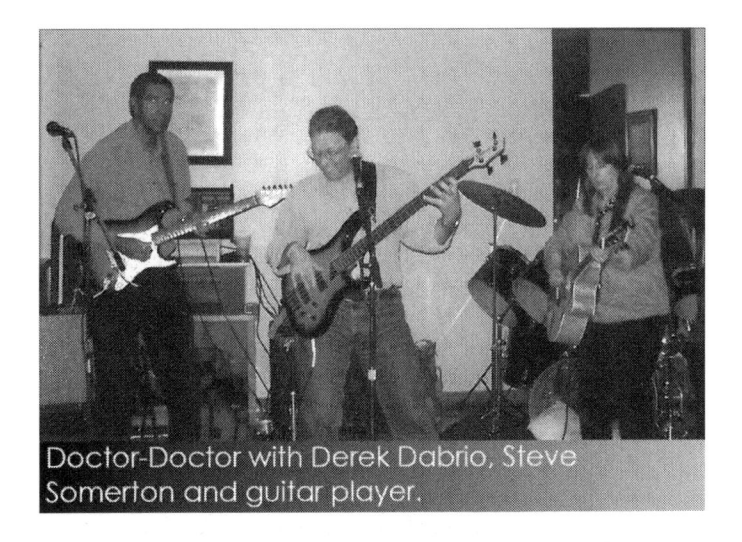

Doctor-Doctor with Derek Dabrio, Steve Somerton and guitar player.

    Later Jackie told me that it gave her a special insight into that side of her sister's life which she wasn't ever aware of.

You have to take a subject like aphasia and see the humour in it. Now that I can laugh again, I can think of any number of funny mix-ups I have been involved in. However, in the early stages of my recovery, I had to rediscover humour.

    For two years after my stroke, I wasn't able to watch television or movies. I just didn't get any jokes that would be based on spoken language. Some of the visual ones still worked though. It is a little better now. I watched the Olympics and began watching Ellen since her show was light and funny without dragging me down.

    The ability to laugh seemed to disappear in that first year. I would listen to people's conversation and what would make others laugh went right by me. When I did start to recover my sense of humour giving me the ability to laugh again, it signified another milestone in my recovery.

    There are also those things you don't miss. I use to be a major nail-biter. I haven't touched them since my stroke.

FUNNY MIX-UPS

Crystal says:	People heard:
Peanut Store	Penis Store
Pudding in the fridge	Pussy in the fridge
You must be a farmer	You must be the farter
Text me	Sex me
My mother hoed (fields)	My mother whored

One thing I really missed was being able to drive. Due to my stroke, I lost my license for one year. That was something I just couldn't understand. Not only did it mean independence for me, being stuck on the farm, not having it meant I would always be dependent on people driving me. I was resolute in my determination to get it back.

In my mind I was still a perfect driver. Today, I know that not being allowed to drive back then was a good thing.

Here is an example of how crazy it would be for me to be driving. In the early days of my recovery as I sat in the back seat of a car driven by others, I would often get confused over what to do with a green light or a red light. "Was it stop or go?"

In hindsight, it was a very good thing that the doctors caring for me didn't agree with me and determined that I should not be driving. In that first year I was only coping...I even had to learn to make pies again. I really wanted to drive again and regain my independence but, the fact of the matter was, driving was not in the cards for me.

However, I was improving gradually and at the end of the year, I was feeling much better. I was sure I could drive but now had to prove that I would be capable of driving.

Waking Up

DRIVING POST-STROKE

Driving is a complex skill. Legally a physician must report any patient who, "is suffering from a condition that may make it dangerous for the person to operate a motor vehicle".
In Crystal's case, she had to wait a minimum of three months to get her license back and still required permission from her physician.

First I had to get permission from my doctors, no easy task. I remember fighting with them to give me a chance and could tell by the way Dr. Devilliers at Hamilton General looked at me that he really didn't think I was ready yet. Still, he heard me out as I was very persistent. At a check-up, he, Jim and Bev were talking about me driving. Once again, I wasn't even part of the conversation, although I was standing in front of them. I stopped them, stood in front of Dr. Devilliers, looked him directly in the eyes and pretended to grab a steering wheel and drive.

It worked. He performed a neurological test designed to test my strength, ability to move and my visual field. Not many people are aware that their visual field will change during a stroke and then also during recovery. Since our brain is an expert in accepting this and compensating, it often goes unnoticed by a stroke victim, yet can be determined by a simple visual test performed by a physician. After a battery of tests he allowed me to go on to the next stage of testing.

I was given another special stroke test in Paris, Ontario to be able to apply for my learner's permit. Although expensive, it was a necessary step. I poured over the learner's permit book but it didn't seem to make sense to me. I got Jim to read it out loud to me just like an interpreter and that worked. He didn't go easy on me, though, while vacationing at the cottage he drilled me constantly.

> **DRIVING RULES*****
>
> Once the physician sends his report to the Ministry of Transportation in Ontario, it is overseen by the Medical Review Section.
>
> **Possible Outcomes:**
> -Immediate suspension
> -Request for additional information
> -Request for an evaluation from a specialist
> -Request for a comprehensive driving evaluation at an approved rehab centre
> -Request for a three part test (vision, written and road test)
> -No action

Since just plain reading of the booklet out loud wasn't effective, (after a few sentences, I just couldn't understand what he was saying), Jim decided to ask me questions. Although it seemed to be effective, it was a frustratingly slow process. Jim, to his credit, toughed it out and we fought on throughout the entire "vacation".

The day that I passed the learner's permit test was huge for me. It was a tremendous relief to finally get a permit that allowed me to practice with someone in the car.

Jim then took me to a parking lot in Norwich and put me through my paces with a test on parallel parking. I was never very good at it before the stroke, so both of us were surprised when I accomplished it perfectly.

Taking the final test was another thing entirely. I didn't have the greatest track record, so to speak. In my first test as a sixteen year old I failed for speeding. In my defense the person in front of me was going really, really slow. I was also driving my dad's new car. One of those beautiful large 70's sedans that floated on its suspension. Driving it at 30 klm. an hour felt like 10 klm. an hour. However, my driving examiner didn't think it was a good enough excuse. Actually I remember him looking a little pale. For my second test I had it all figured out but going slower didn't seem to work any better than speeding. I failed again.

All this was on my mind when we pulled up to the Driver Examination Centre in Paris. 37 years later, I knew I would have to re-live the experience all over again.

I was ready to go and sat there, nervously waiting behind the steering wheel. Finally, two people got in the back of the car and the examiner took his position in the front. That only increased my anxiety. I didn't understand why the two people in the back were there. And then they started to talk, and talk, and talk. I managed to keep my focus on the road and not on their conversation.

The two were a psychologist and a nurse testing my ability to concentrate. It was all part of the test and this time I was much more successful than my first three attempts when I was sixteen.

Getting my license back was a real milestone in my

> **POSSIBILITY OF DRIVING**
>
> 30 to 40 % of individuals who experience a stroke resume driving. The best predictors of driving outcome appear to be vision, cognition, driving experience and functional ability.
>
> The more experience an individual has driving, the more automatic his/her actions become.
>
> *Heart and Stroke Foundation Ontario Stroke System*

recovery. My greatest joy today is driving with no-one in the car. That way there is no talking to have to deal with, just pure freedom.

    I worked hard with Jan on some special phrases that would help me in my driving experiences. Most importantly, when I pull up to the Tim Hortons drive-through now, I try to speak each word clearly into the microphone. "Large coffee with milk...No thanks, I don't want anything else. Thank you." If they get it, I leave them a tip. If not, I end up going inside to make them understand.

12 THE TRUTH IN "GIVING BACK"

As I began to feel better, both mentally and physically, I began to do a fair bit of travelling. Frequently I would go with my sister Kim, to visit Jackie, who lives in LA. Knowing me, Jackie only set one ground rule for my visits, telling me in no uncertain terms, "Crystal - if you see anyone famous, you are not going to approach them."

However, one good thing about a stroke is that you can always blame your behaviour on your condition.

One day, Jackie and I had gone out for lunch. On the way there, while looking across the street, someone caught my eye. They had stepped into a local post office. Crossing the street, I casually looked into the window and saw that my hunch was right. It was the actress, Jamie Lee Curtis, whom I've always wanted to meet.

Meanwhile, Jackie figured out what I was up to. She let me know that there was no way she was going to go up to the star as she was too embarrassed. I told her, "I'm not," and entered the Post Office before Jackie could stop me.

I managed to tell the tall and fit woman, "I'm not from here, I want to say hi." She asked me where I was from and by that time I had reached the extent of my language abilities and spilled out, "not talk right - aneurysm." She stopped right there and it was just me and her. She asked me questions and I responded. I don't remember the specifics of the conversation but I remember it being very heartfelt and honest.

When she found out my sister was outside waiting with her dog, Jamie opened the door, stepped outside and introduced herself saying, "I just met your sister, she is an amazing person." She was very generous and at the end of our conversation Jamie hugged me tightly and her parting words were, "You are super courageous."

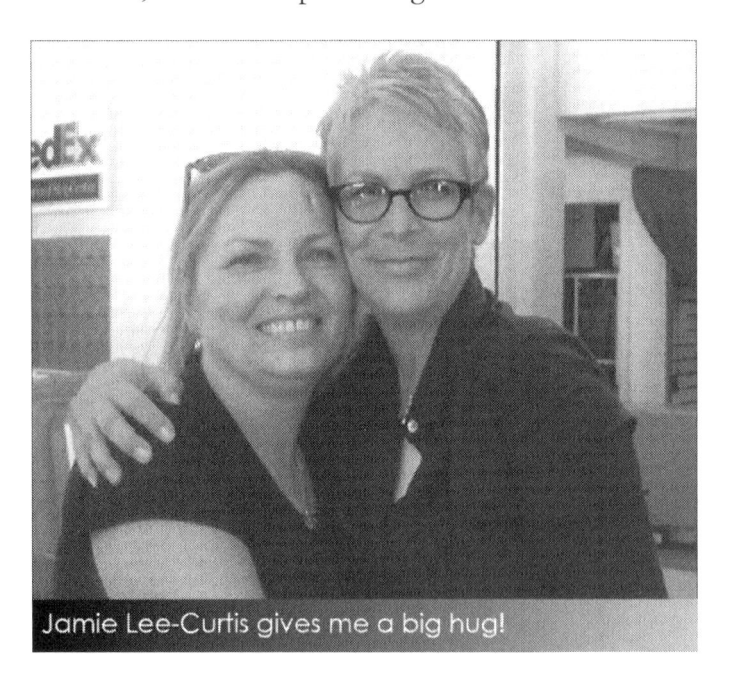

Jamie Lee-Curtis gives me a big hug!

I also met James Caan. While going out to dinner at Mr. Chow in Beverly Hills, camera flashes began going off behind us. We looked around and saw it was the famous actor. I was a bit taken back by how tall he was, but not having the ability to speak had never stopped me before. It wasn't going to stop me now. Before Jackie had a chance to

Waking Up

grab me, I walked up to him. He looked at me curiously as I made it past his bodyguard. "Stroke," I stammered. "Love your movies..." I showed him my camera and said, "picture?"

He stopped me, smiled, took my camera and gave it to his bodyguard. Then he slipped his big masculine arm around me and had his bodyguard take a couple of pictures. He was very gracious.

For some reason, I got it in my head that we had to go give a gift to Ellen DeGeneres. I love Ellen. She was a constant companion in my days at home, slowly recovering. Hers was a show that I was able to watch and understand. Trying to re-learn how to talk, and practicing with her in front of the television, she seemed like a real friend to me.

When we got to the studio, I gathered my gifts together. I was giving her a letter I had written, a bottle of Wayne Gretzky Estate Wine and a Blue Rodeo CD. I told my sisters to wait in the car. They were not too happy with letting the person with aphasia do the negotiations so they wanted to deliver it. To their credit they knew me and could see how determined I was. I carefully explained, "Call if need you."

I strolled up to the doorman and started explaining why I was there. "Saw...him, television...positive." The more I attempted to communicate, the more frustrated I became. Not a good combination for a stroke victim. Finally, my beautiful sisters came to my rescue and let him know what I was trying to say. We were successful and the gift went in to Ellen (I'm still waiting for my thank you card).

In the third year of my stroke recovery, I took a trip to Beverly Hills. On arriving at the airport, I anxiously searched for my sister, Jackie who was picking me up. Again, just like a baby I had only re-learned a few words.

At the airline terminal I was under the handicap watch and forced to use a wheelchair. That just didn't sit well with me since my legs were fine. As they wheeled me past the other passengers waiting to get picked up, I felt like I was on display. Despite being capable of thinking in my mind, here I was, back in my stroller again.

The harsh reality was that I was still a stroke victim and had to submit to being treated like a newborn. I did have one little victory though. After reassuring the attendant that I was fine, she turned around. I then got up and walked to the bathroom. Returning, I sat back in the chair and looking at the other passenger's bemused looks, I saw the humour in it.

There is a point when you have to state your own independence to your loved ones. In Haliburton, my friend and I went to get a facial. I had no license at the time and had to be driven everywhere and it was getting to me. When we entered the shop, my friend, as usual, stepped in front of me to tell the woman what I wanted done. I had enough of being looked after and I purposely stepped in front of her to give my own instructions, saying, "I will talk myself."

I felt good that I was taking my life back. From my experience, I would say that stroke is all about that. Reclaiming your life back every day.

THE MIRACLE

I kept flashing back to Dr. Dabreo's statement, "Crystal, you are a miracle!" Since I began my recovery I had been searching for ways to positively affect others around with my "miracle." The opportunity came to me when a prominent physician invited Kim and I out to lunch.

Dr. Richard Johnson, Chief of Staff at the Brantford General, met us in the beautiful wood-grained lobby of the Brantford Golf and Country Club. As we approached the table, I was surprised to see a large group of people seated there. Dr. Johnson introduced me to members of the Brant Community Healthcare System Foundation, most of whom I knew already through my previous work at the Hospital.

He got to the point and told me they wanted me to lead the staff fund-raising campaign.

> **VOLUNTEERING****
>
> Once you achieve a level of comfort with family and friends, if possible, you can volunteer. Helping others often helps you feel better about yourself. Remember there is no rush and you should step into this stage at a comfortable pace.

I knew that I had helped the Foundation before, but this was now. I was no longer the person I was pre-stroke and I questioned their choice of leader. Dr. Johnson insisted that he knew I could do it. A wise doctor he was since it is good for recovering stroke patients to keep active socially.

It was the beginning of many adventures for me and as part of my new responsibilities, I had to gather gifts for the next Foundation special event. My sister Kim, knowing how important this was to me and my recovery, graciously agreed to help out by driving me around.

One of the first places I approached was the Pinestone Resort, Conference Centre and Golf Course. I knew the manager and they had donated a weekend stay the previous year so I was pretty sure they would do so again. When I arrived I was disappointed at my bad timing since Cynthia, the previous manager had left for parts unknown and I didn't recognize the new man's name.

As I was leaving, I saw a man in a suit who looked to be in charge. I asked him if he was the new manager, and that was when I met Frank Vismeg. He introduced himself and smiling, shook my hand.

By that time it was later in the day and I had reached my limits. I was exhausted trying to ask for the manager, I was exhausted explaining what I wanted and I was just plain exhausted. I struggled to hold them back yet tears found

their way into my eyes.
Frank showed me into his office and gently sat me down. He ordered me a coffee and handed me a Kleenex. Determined to get my message out and seeing that I had his total attention, I dried my tears and set about my task.

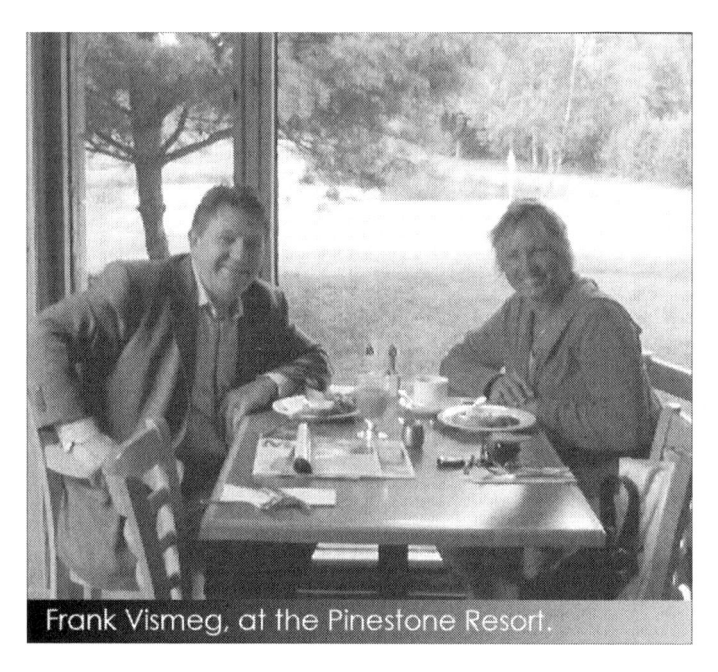

Frank Vismeg, at the Pinestone Resort.

Armed with determination and courage, I struggled to make myself understood. In the end he found out what I was asking for and I presented the foundation with a two night, all-inclusive weekend at the resort.

Frank was so nice about my break-down that I had to bake him a pie. We brought the pie and a bottle of Wayne Gretzky Estate wine to him the next day. Did I mention that I am not shy? I got Frank to throw in an extra breakfast as part of the package. Like the word in Jim Cuddy's song, the key to coping with aphasia is to keep trying. Sometimes it works out.

When I arrived at the large company in Brantford, S.C.

Johnson, the person at the reception desk was blind. I quickly realized that my usual routine of writing and drawing pictures was not going to work.

However he was incredibly patient and accommodating, listening and trying to ask the right questions. After some monumental efforts on both our parts, I came out with a donation.

The night of the big Foundation event came and hundreds of people gathered in the ballroom at the Brant Park Inn. Along with my fellow nurse and long-time friend Marlyn Usher and the ever-present Kim, I had to get up in front of donors and give a speech. It was to be my first time speaking in public after my stroke.

I felt like a baby again as I stumbled over my words. I had learned one special phrase for my speech, "Thank you. I hope you enjoyed the wine." I managed to get that out and make it through the night with the help of my friends.

> **FATIGUE STRATEGIES**
>
> People who have had a stroke may become fatigued quite easily. An analogy would be a cast on a wrist. When unwrapped from the cast, the limb is weak and shriveled. It requires a combination of rest and rehabilitation. For the stroke victim it is the same, except it affects the entire body. This is a normal process. Allow yourself time to nap or sleep when you need it.
>
> *Dr. Thorsteinn Gunnarson, Neurologist*

Later that evening, Dr. Johnson stepped up to the podium and began his speech to wrap things up. Mentioning me, the esteemed doctor gave me a clue that I was doing well with my recovery when he said at the podium, "Thank God for giving Crystal back to us. She is an inspiration to all of us."

A year later when he retired as Chief of Staff and a new CEO took over the hospital, Marlyn and I thought it was the perfect time to move on. Dr. Johnson was the reason that we got involved in the first place. He made it all a success because of his inclusive personality. Whether you worked in nutrition services, the operating room, the pharmacy or Tim Hortons, he treated all equally.

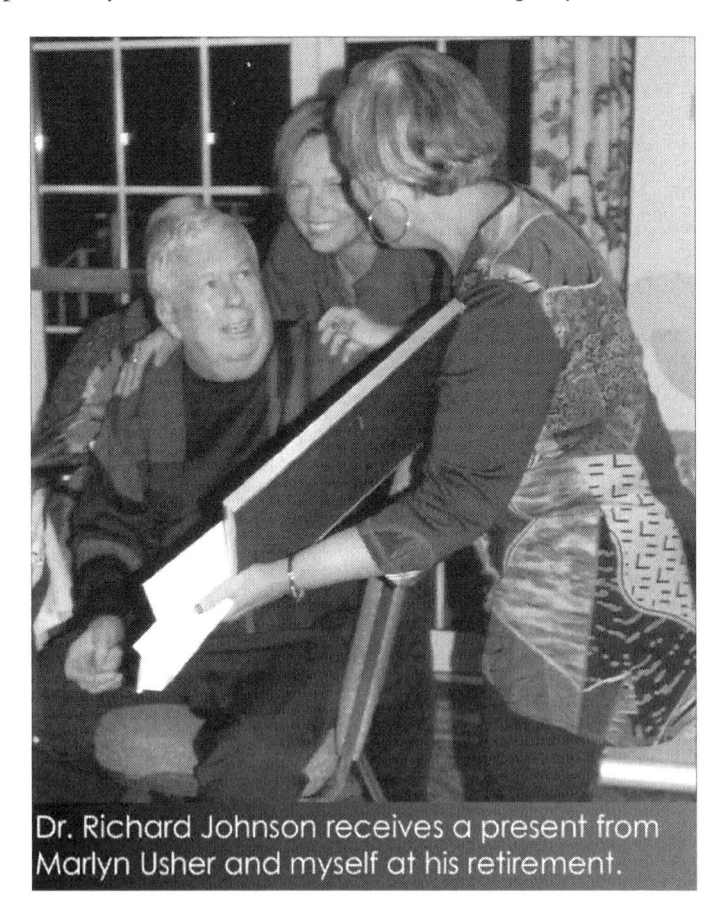

Dr. Richard Johnson receives a present from Marlyn Usher and myself at his retirement.

His quiet and powerful demeanor inspired people across

the hospital to give up their time and donate to the Hospital Foundation. He also did it in a way that made the world around him casual and fun.

When I spoke at one of the Hospital Foundation events, I meant it when I said, "I know he helped the hospital but I will always be grateful for how he helped me."

I had many proud moments while I was volunteering at the Foundation that would not have occurred if my life had taken a different path without the stroke. Curious how life can take something profound away, yet still give back at the same time.

13 MAKING A NEW LIFE

As I continue to slowly make my way forward to a new normal, I realize that life can be a never-ending story. A couple of years ago, I thought my book was finished and began a search for a publisher. Unfortunately life got in the way and when we returned to it, the story wasn't complete anymore.

We needed to work on new chapters of the book since some of my experiences lately might be of benefit to stroke survivors. Suffice it to say that every day now I look for a new chapter since we may not be here tomorrow.

Post-recovery I realize that I am not the same person I used to be. Although I used to be an early riser, my stroke has made me a really early riser. I now regularly wake up at 4:30 in the morning and rarely make it past 9 in the evening.

Despite my speech difficulties, I forget that I have aphasia sometimes. Kelly laughs when she tells the story of being stopped for speeding. She was bringing me home from a hospital appointment when she was pulled over. As the officer came to the window, I proceeded to tell her that Kelly was just bringing me home from the hospital and we promised to never speed again. All this in my nonsense language. Noticing the puzzled look on the officer's face, Kelly turned to me and gave me a very forceful, "Crystal!

Shhh." The officer proceeded to write her the ticket anyway.

Sadly, I have had to say goodbye to a good friend and colleague who, in so many ways, is responsible for my recovery. After, Jan left the Brantford General Hospital, we lost touch for a few months. I realized that I wanted her to be part of my life and see her again, so I tracked her down. I finally located her and arranged to meet at the Blue Dog, a coffee shop near the hospital.

As we talked I found out about how her life had changed. She was still working with patients although she had slowed down a bit. She told me she had cancer but the treatments seemed to be working and it was in remission. She then floored me by offering to pay for a trip for a month to Halifax so that I could work on an intensive speech therapy program.

I was torn between going and staying but a trip to the Maritimes was not to be. During that period, both Mrs. White and Dr. White had been diagnosed with cancer. I wanted to be there for them and see them both through their therapy. Sadly, Jan's cancer came back a year later and that day at the cafe was the last time I would see her alive. I miss her so much.

ROAD TO RECOVERY

"In a stroke, some parts of the brain may be damaged and other parts may be simply stunned and will recover. Typically, recovery will be rapid over the first six months and slower over the next two years. At the end of that period, it is likely that is as far as your recovery will go."
Dr. Thorsteinn Gunnarson, Neurologist

In recovery we have to re-invent ourselves. I know I can never return to nursing as a career but I am acutely aware

Waking Up

that I still have talents in this area. I also know how great the responsibility is in nursing hands and I always make sure I have assistance.

A neighbour down the road at the White's cottage asked me to help with a needle since he needed a vitamin B12 injection. I agreed, but only if my sister Kim and my sister-in-law, Bev were present. That way both nurses could check that the dosage I was giving was correct. I have to admit, it was like old times when I gave the needle. I hadn't lost my nursing touch.

Nursing experiences seem to keep looking for me. On my way home one day, I noticed a perfect table and chair in the style that my neighbour had been looking for. Since I am not shy, I went up to the older lady sitting on her porch and asked her if I could buy them from her. She didn't quite understand what I was saying but allowed me to take them away. I left her my name and number telling her in my halting English that if there was anything I could do for her all she had to do was call.

At 6:30 the next morning the phone rang. It was the lady sitting on the porch and she had called me as I invited her to. She had lost her glasses and wanted me to go into her optometrist to order a replacement. The next morning she called again with a question about the war. I went over to see her but couldn't quite understand why the war would be still affecting her. I listened and tried to be sympathetic.

Over the next week she called me daily but I still couldn't get clear what she was telling me. Finally her son called me to ask about her medications. What I thought were questions about the war were really questions about the medication warfarin. It turns out that she thought I was the VON nurse! Once a nurse, always a nurse I guess.

Another time, I was baby-sitting my grandson, James Hunter Courtland-White, or Hunter as he is known. He was heavily into teething and his mother asked me to give him some Tylenol. Keenly aware of my limitations, I had her measure out the dosage before she left.

Often, I can make my stroke work for me and have a good time doing it. My sisters and I went shopping one afternoon at Costco. I spied an item on the top shelf. Although they had been told that employees can't get things down from the top shelf, I smiled and told my sisters that wasn't going to stop me. They looked at each other with that look that said, "Oh no, what is Crystal going to get us into now?"

Winking at them, I called a man who worked there over. I pointed to the item on the top shelf and explained, "try shop, can't, stroke stroke". I was just about on the verge of pulling my tears out when he relented and pulled the item down for me. I felt a little guilty but it was a victory and it seemed to entertain my sisters.

My family has adjusted to life with me and continue to help me out. One of the things I still have difficulty understanding is my cell phone bill. Actually, this may not be due to my stroke, since I have heard the same thing from many people who don't have strokes! However, it is really difficult for me to follow bills so my son James always checks them over to see if I am reading them correctly before I pay them.

Using a cell phone doesn't seem to be a problem for me, but retrieving messages can be difficult and rewarding. I can understand what people are saying, but hearing and understanding numbers was almost impossible at the beginning stages of my recovery. My understanding of numbers has slowly improved but it takes me a long time to write out a phone number. When I first started answering messages after my stroke, I had to repeat each message at least ten times to get it right. Today, I only have to repeat it five or six times. I have to really focus on listening when I talk on the phone as the fine details are easy to miss.

Another issue that has to be confronted are the financial implications that come with a stroke. While in Buffalo, we incurred significant roaming fees. These mounted up into the thousands of dollars. While recovering, I remember laying tired in bed, listening to Jim getting bullied by the carrier to pay our bills. I was thankful that Jim didn't give into them. He is a strong person and wasn't going to let them have their way.

The silver lining here is brain training. I know that it is good exercise for me to listen to and write out numbers. Texting is something I am good at but I honestly don't like it and will only do it when necessary. I would rather hear a person's voice as it helps me understand better.

I am working on improving my use of technology. For instance, debit cards are an everyday fact of life for most people. I have had one for over twenty years now and before my stroke, I never thought twice about it, using it daily. I remember the first time I tried to use one after my stroke. For the life of me, I couldn't remember the number and it brought me to tears. Later we found the number in my files at home. I have worked hard to re-learn that skill but my need to shop for bargains has helped inspire me.

Although my relationship with debit cards has improved, I still need help sometimes. A note to all family members of stroke victims, please feel free to offer your assistance when you see us struggling with an ATM.

BANKING TIPS

-If you have regular income like disability payments or pensions set up direct deposit and you can avoid difficulties with deposits.
-With regular bill payments, set up automatic withdrawals to ensure they get paid.
-Identify a trusted family member and have their name added to your bank account. That way they can help you and also monitor banking activity on your account

Waking Up

It may be hard to see them but there are a few silver linings to the effects of a stroke. Prior to my stroke, I would bribe my co-workers with coffee to work on the computer for me, since I was really techno-phobic. Now, I have had time to learn how to use a basic computer. My niece, Ali was working for a computer company and she got me my first computer.

I remember distinctly when I finally learned to use e-mail. Kim called me and we began talking over the phone. I stumbled and couldn't find a word. As my frustration grew, she told me to go upstairs and turn on the computer. My wonderful sister walked me through everything and soon, I was communicating with her over the computer by e-mail. It actually worked. Interestingly, I was not able to say the word over the phone but the moment I sat down at the keyboard, I could type it. Her e-mail lesson was more of gift than she will ever know.

We all have to keep moving forward. Today, I have a speech therapy technique that I have developed myself that personifies this and keeps the conversation going. If I have to repeat myself more than three times, I say, "forget it," and move on. This works for me and everyone else.

14 THE NEXT CHAPTER

Today, my life is changing once again as Jim and I have now sold the farm in Hatchley. We have also decided to go our separate ways. When we bought the farm I was a country girl and Jim was a city boy with a passion for farming. Together we accomplished a lot.

Ending a relationship is a little like surgery. There is cutting, pain and healing involved. Whether we would have separated if I had not had a stroke, who can say?

DIVORCE/SEPARATION

In a study done on the National Health Institute Survey in the United States in 1999, it was determined people with spouses that were disabled were much more likely to be divorced or separated at 20.7 percent, while only 13.1 percent of the households had been through a divorce without any disability as a factor.

It became apparent when we decided to "sell the farm." We had been together for 36 years, so the idea came as a bit of a shock to everyone in the family. I guess that it was

Waking Up

something that had been building between us. For two years prior there were signs that we were growing apart. Jim and I had just celebrated our 33rd year of marriage and I was feeling extremely grateful to have had him as my husband.

Honestly, I may have seen it coming but I always held out hope that we could work it out. The idea of us separating, well that rocked me to the core. After a few years of trying to work it out it became apparent that the two of us could no longer remain together and we both moved on.

Since our separation I now live in a small but comfortable bungalow in Brantford and Jim continues his life elsewhere. Who knows where it will go and what can one say about divorce? I feel like it is going to take me some time to heal from it. Last Christmas, my new home felt a little more empty without the farmhouse and normal family life. Despite not being together, to this day, I still depend on Jim and know he will be there if I need him.

However, my boys and their families all live close by and we visit frequently. The greatest joy of my life is being involved in my boy's families.

Although my right leg still drags when I am tired, and to this day, nine years after my stroke, I still mix up "he" and "she", I now feel safe looking after my grandson. I have to be careful when running a bath for him since I still can't trust the feeling in my right hand so I make sure to test the warmth of the water for the little one with my left hand.

One of my greatest accomplishments during my recovery has been the long journey to finally look after him. I say I look after him but it really is a two way street.

Coincidentally, my current speech therapist is my grandson, Hunter. We get together every week or more. Although he is young, it works for me. As a toddler, I started by sitting him down and reading stories from his books. However, having a toddler as a therapist had its draw backs since he didn't have a lot of patience.

The next stage in my therapy session usually involved spending a lot of time chasing him. As I ran after him, I read him books on the run and tried to make him understand me. I'm not sure how successful I am but he seems to like his crazy grandmother.

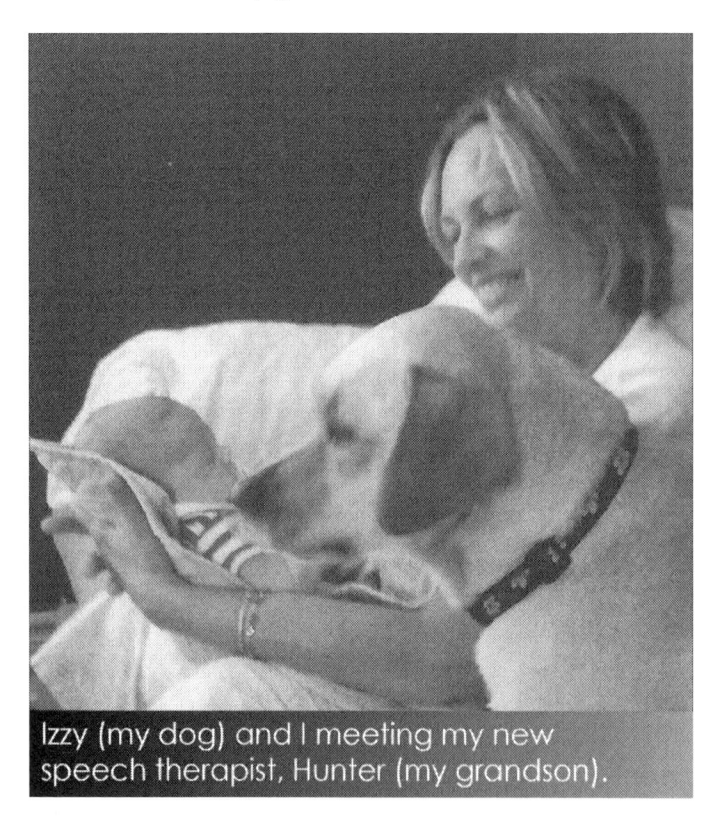

Izzy (my dog) and I meeting my new speech therapist, Hunter (my grandson).

I have a new appreciation for little people because of my aphasia. My son Chase' girlfriend's name is Amanda. When Hunter was two and a half, he heard me trying to say her name and it was coming out, "Manana." He said to me, "You are not saying it right," and proceeded to correct me each time I said her name until I got it right. I thought to myself, "Oh my God, he has learned this and is now teaching me." I still carry that precious memory with me.

Waking Up

Every day I count my blessings as I return to this "circle of life." I still do my own speech therapy every morning, reading, and practicing speaking out loud. Keeping at it has helped me. However, there are some things I, and my family, just have to accept with a sense of humour. Since I stumble over some words such as my son Chase's name, I think we may have permanently changed it to Ch...ch...chase."

There are symptoms of my stroke that will likely persist. As a nurse I learned about "footdrop". This is a term for difficulty lifting the front part of the foot. If you have foot drop, you may drag the front of your foot on the ground when you walk.

Foot drop isn't a disease. Rather, foot drop is a sign of an neurological or muscular problem. Sometimes foot drop is temporary. Or in other cases such as mine, foot drop is permanent. If you have foot drop, you may need to wear a brace on your ankle and foot to hold your foot in a normal position. Although it isn't as severe as when I first began recovery, I still use a pillow to position it in the proper position when I am tired and laying down.

I hope this book about my journey helps to give you an insight into waking up in the world of stroke and aphasia. We must move on and after all, any of us could face losing our voices or have a family member lose their voice. In retrospect, I realize that it was not just my life that changed with my stroke but it affected the lives of all the people connected to me.

Understanding that you are going through this process and meeting the challenges of a stroke victim's recovery together with your family members is the best way to get your life back. Don't ever give up and try to keep a positive attitude. After all, how many people get a second chance to wake up? Every day I am grateful just to wake up healthy.

I still feel that my Dad is watching over me and my grandmother's words ring in my ears when I get down,

"Your dad is watching and he wouldn't want to see you sad!"

    Today, as I unpack my things, I remember the sunset on the back porch in Hatchley and think about how I am going to miss it. But life always changes and there are two sides to every coin. Moving on sometimes means just exchanging one sunset for another. With much hope!

Waking Up

ABOUT THE AUTHOR

Peter Muir is a writer, director and photographer living in Port Dover Ontario. He is Artistic Director of the Bell Summer Theatre Festival and has written a number of plays and film scripts including his latest book, Brantford General Hospital, 125 Years of Caring. Working for a number of years at the Brant Community Healthcare System he and Crystal became friends and he is pleased to be able to tell Crystal's story.